Blind Man Running

*A Product of the Ozark Mountains-The Story of a
Blind Man's Quest for the Joy of Life*

by
Michael McIntire

Bloomington, IN Milton Keynes, UK

authorHOUSE™

AuthorHouse™
1663 Liberty Drive, Suite 200
Bloomington, IN 47403
www.authorhouse.com
Phone: 1-800-839-8640

AuthorHouse™ UK Ltd.
500 Avebury Boulevard
Central Milton Keynes, MK9 2BE
www.authorhouse.co.uk
Phone: 08001974150

Library of Congress Control Number: 2006902180

First published by AuthorHouse 4/12/2006

ISBN: 1-4259-2255-4 (sc)

Printed in the United States of America
Bloomington, Indiana

This book is printed on acid-free paper.
Cover photo by Sandie Zemblidge

Reviews

"I have also been involved in the music business; and when I met Michael McIntire I was impressed by his music and his spirit. Michael is a wonderful person with a great story to tell. His book is entitled "Blind Man Running" and there couldn't be a more fitting title to describe his approach to life. One remark in his book, "I may be blind, but I have vision", is so fitting to Michael as a person, whom you will discover in his book, has a tremendous amount of vision and ambition. His story talks about his trials and tribulations as a youngster growing up, with all the normal inquisitiveness, and dealing with it while having a limited amount of eyesight, of which he never let be an obstacle. It may have made things interesting, but never impossible. The book will take you through Michael's life and entertain you with all his experiences told in such a refreshing and entertaining style, including many emotions and his personal insight.

Michael, who is an accomplished musician/singer/songwriter, lets nothing hold him back from pursuing his dreams. He truly is an inspiration, and I am sure that reading his book will do nothing but entertain and inspire you.

Take a trip with "Blind Man Running" and hold on for the ride!"
Gale Walh Kelliher, Saskatchewan Canada

"Read this book and you will get to know a man who lives life to the fullest. Michael writes from the heart. He has experienced adventure, danger and love. He enables the reader to travel with him and become part of the action. I couldn't stop reading!"
Anne Guelker
St. Louis, Missouri

"These pages will keep you on the edge of your seat as you wait to read the outcome of events in Michael's world. Being blind myself, I can relate to a lot of the frustrations he faces and commend him for speaking out. I thoroughly enjoyed his writing and believe me; you will not regret purchasing this book."
Stephie Bell
Auckland, New Zealand

"This is a wonderful book about life, which will be appreciated by all who take the time to read it. Michael McIntire is not only an incredible musician, but a fantastic story teller who brings his unique prospective on life as a blind, traveling musician to great story after great story! He will make you laugh, think, and appreciate so many things that you take for granted every day."
Kyle Everett
St. Louis, Missouri

"All I can say is WOW, has this guy got one heck of a story or what?! I didn't intend to read the whole thing at once, but when it is that good…you can't help yourself."
Anthony Reno
Roberts Recording Studio
West Plains, Missouri

Acknowledgments

I would like to thank my publisher, Ron Bowles, for his patience and understanding; my old buddy, Marlin Knight, for technical support, along with his great sense of humor; my editor, Gordon Johnston, for helping me keep my literary ducks in a row; and last but certainly not least, my lady, Sandie, for being there every step of the way.

Dedication

This book is dedicated to Nina Juanita McIntire.
When I had fallen, she helped me stand.
When my life was broken, she was there to pick up the pieces.
Thanks Mom.

Chapter 1
Hide and Seek

My story begins in St. Louis, Missouri on February 25, 1950. When I was around two we moved to a house on the South Side. The address was 1754 Simpson Place, off of LaFayette Street, just a block from Lafayette Park. Isn't it odd how you can remember your address as a child or your phone number (Prospect 1 2498), but it's so hard to remember what you had for dinner last night? I vividly recollect getting chased out of that park by street gangs. Of course they were tame compared to modern gangs. To me they were quite real. I would run from the park looking over my shoulder, eyes wide with sheer terror. They were relentless. I would dart out into traffic, taking my chances with an automobile weighing thousands of pounds and squashing me like a bug rather than suffer a bloody nose from one of those little punks who, in reality, were probably no tougher than I was. Now I am an adult so I no longer do silly things such as that. I have an extensive list of silly things that I practice on a daily basis.

I was a normal child doing things that kids do. If I had limitations I was unaware of them. Little did I know what was just around the corner! For the rest of my life, friends, relatives, teachers, and people I worked with would be more than happy to make me painfully aware of what they thought my limitations should be. I am grateful to God that when he bestowed blindness upon me he also gave me the gift of spirit. I am fond of saying, "I may be blind but I have vision." I promise there will be more tasty morsels of wit and wisdom thrown to you throughout this book.

My first recollection of having a problem with my eyesight was while playing hide and seek. (I still play that game occasionally when the woman will participate.) One night we were playing in the alley. I was running for home base at full speed. At that time I could distinguish shadows. I was running down the alley in the shadow of a garage when all of a sudden I felt intense pain in my arm. It seems there was a water faucet that had jumped from the garage to make it known to me, and boy, did it ever. My arm was sore the next day. That was only the beginning. I was to have many bumps and bruises over the years from things that my eyes could not see. (I-44 now runs through the house where I lived until I was around eleven. The alley still runs adjacent to it.) At that time my sight was pretty good. I could still see stars and planets at night; however, more and more I noticed that I could not do things that other kids could do. For instance, when a ball was thrown to me I would have a hard time tracking it with my vision; so many times I would miss it.

I was in third grade when the school sent a note home to my mother. Apparently my visual deterioration had begun. They recommended a specialist, and after an examination I was diagnosed with "retinitis pigmentosa", a hereditary eye disease of the retina. It affects the cells of the retina which take in light. It is carried by the female. (Consequently I have spent a lifetime trying unsuccessfully to convince my mother that it was not her fault.)

I had two uncles who were afflicted with this disease. They raised families, held jobs, and most of all, did not indulge in self pity. I like to think that I inherit my good humor about my blindness from them. That's right! I said blindness, not visually impaired, not handicapped, not disabled, or any of that other politically correct bullshit. I remember a few years ago some national blind organizations were raising a stink about the movie, *Mr. Magoo*. The main character was a blind guy who went around barely escaping catastrophe. Somehow I can relate. DUH! Did you notice that political correctness gets me fired up somewhat?

I am certain that at some point during my childhood the seed of denial was sown. We all participated—me, my parents, my friends, and my relatives. We were all experts at denial. I have to say that if I had it to do all over I wouldn't change a thing. You say, "But why? They could have sent you to a special blind school." Yeah, they would put you in your place, all right. They could teach you how to be blind. I was pretty good at that, thank you very much. It's my opinion that in public schools of any kind there is a certain degree of brainwashing that takes place. Yeah, I was in denial, but as time went on I adapted to the situations I found myself in. Hell, by the time I graduated from high school only a handful of kids in my inner circle knew how poor my eyesight was. My skills in denial would really come into play later. Like everyone else, I was in preparation as a child for my life as an adult.

Despite my blindness my childhood was fairly uneventful. The real fun would come later, as my ego developed and my hormones raged.

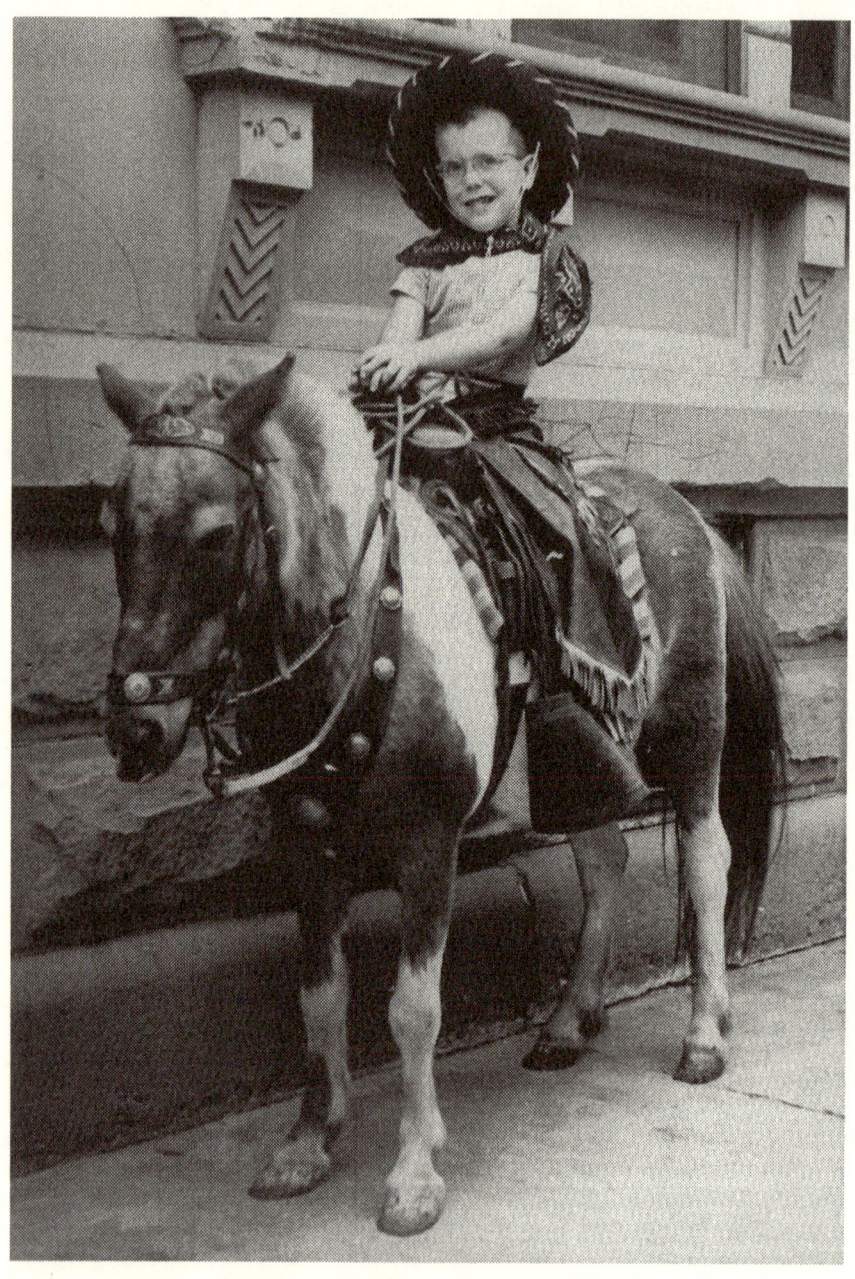

Michael at approximately age 4
Nickelson Avenue, across from Lafayette Park, Saint Louis, MO

Chapter 2
Country Life

When I was twelve my parents decided it was time for the family to go into business.

We moved to Eminence, a small town in the Ozarks in south central Missouri. We bought some land just north of town on Highway 19 and built the Riverside, a motel which is still in business today. The move could have had no less effect on me if my father had loaded the family into a space ship and taken us to Mars. Don't get me wrong, I loved the country and still do. Some of my fondest memories as a child are of visiting my grandparents for Christmas and of fishing, swimming, and boating on the Jack's Fork and Current Rivers in the summer. I was a twelve-year-old stranger in a strange land. In the big city of St. Louis I was already going to sock-hops, wearing slacks, and shining my shoes. Oh yeah, there was a thing called "girls." I remember coming home from my new school after having been there just three days and begging my mother to "please buy me some tennis shoes and jeans."

At this time my eye disease had progressed very little, but my general anxiety was warming up its engines for the fun that was soon to arrive.

Up until then, like most children, I didn't stray far from home. I was surrounded by the love and protection of my immediate family. It was a big, wide, wonderful world out there, and nothing was going to stop me from experiencing as much of it as I could. Not even poor eyesight would slow me down. Hell, what poor eyesight? I was still in denial and would be for years to come.

When I was in the eighth grade they changed the color of blackboards to green. I don't know what that was about, but suddenly I could see nothing of what the teacher was writing. Also, I couldn't read textbooks for more than ten minutes without suffering from eye fatigue. I know now that I should have brought this to the attention of my teachers, although I am not sure they could or would have helped me. One must remember this was the early '60s. Around this time I was starting to think of myself as Mr. Cool. (Some things haven't changed.) I was wearing Beatle boots, black leather jackets, and a jelly-roll hairdo that would stop traffic. If you look in my yearbook you will see that they gave me the dubious distinction of "boy with the most outstanding hairdo."

To reveal a weakness, especially poor eyesight, to my classmates or teachers is something Mr. Cool could never do. I would sooner have given birth to a porcupine backwards than to wind up in "special education" or another alternative that would prove to be equally un-cool. From the time I was in the third grade I had been hearing sweet little comments from girls. Things like, "Michael would be really cute if he just didn't wear glasses." It's no wonder that if you look at early pictures of me from grade school through college and beyond you will see no frames on this mug. When asked about this I would quip, "Man, I wasn't born with glasses, and I'm not going to have my picture taken with them."

Once, I read about my eye disease in a medical book. Guess what? Right there in print it said that "a common symptom of retinitis pigmentosa is neurosis." That must mean that I started my trip down "insane alley" as a child. At the time of this great medical insight I was in my thirties. By this time I was one of the most cynical bastards you could ever hope to meet. I remember thinking at the time, "All right, now I have an excuse, I can get away with anything. I'm sorry judge, I'm crazy, just look in the medical books."

In the ninth grade things started to get interesting. I was straying further away from the family unit. It was around this time that I started to get curious about life as an adult. For instance getting drunk! What was it like? I had been watching adults drink for years. Why did they do it? It must be fun. Once I saw my uncle pass out on the carport in the middle of the afternoon. I thought to myself, "Wow, he must be tired." I didn't know he was drunk. What fun he was having!

Anyway, some of my friends and I decided to have a go at it. We decided to go camping. Was this not what all-American children should do? Explore the great outdoors? Yeah, I would explore it all right, on my hands and knees.

It was a great plan. For months we saved our money, made lists of necessary items such as camping gear, food, and oh yes, let's not forget the whiskey, a fifth for each of us. To this day, when I smell or taste Seagram's Seven I think of that camping expedition. This was the plan—after dinner we would sit around the fire and with our bottles in hand, find out what it was like to be an adult and get shit-faced.

We devoured an excellent meal, washed dishes, and were ready to pick the evil fruit from the tree. We broke the seal and took the first drink. I quickly learned why the Indians called it fire water. Of course we were careful to keep a straight face. After all, were we not men? Had we not successfully run the river in our canoes without soaking our bed clothes? We had arrived against all odds, and now "by god, we were gonna drink like the big boys."

Each swallow went down easier than the last. Within ten minutes we were on our journey to adulthood. At some point it had turned into a race. We asked each other, "How much you got left?" At this point in our lives we had not heard of the term alcohol poisoning, but I doubt if it would have made much difference anyway, 'cause we were men. As you can imagine, from then on I don't remember much. It was the first but not the last time I would be blind drunk. I know that I didn't make it to the bottom of my bottle. There was close to an inch of whiskey left. It was there, taunting me: "C'mon you're almost there, you're almost a man."

This would be the first situation in which I would find myself in danger and that my blindness would not allow my escape. It was like a dream. I could hear raised voices. There was scuffling. At this point in my life I could see to drive or run a canoe down the river during daylight, but when the sun went down I could only see light from street lamps, headlights on a car, campfires, etc. Suddenly I saw stars, and then I was flat on my back. I felt shock, confusion, and tremendous pain. The pain was quickly replaced by fear. Slowly I began to realize what had happened. Someone had struck me right between the eyes. Instinctively I began to crawl away from the point of danger. I could see absolutely nothing, but I could hear someone crawling behind me. I lost it. I turned and climbed on top of this person and began pounding his head with my fists. Now I know this sounds brutal, but remember I had just drunk a bottle of whiskey. I just wanted to render my assailant helpless so I could get the hell out of there. Until that moment I had not known such fear. I am certain that my blindness played its ghastly role in this nightmare. I managed to crawl for a distance of thirty yards or so before losing consciousness beneath a bluff.

The next day I awoke in the leaves. It was cold, and overcast in more ways than one. I staggered back to camp. Everything was hurting—my head, my stomach, and most of all, my nose. I made my way to the end of the boat to splash some cold river water on my face, thinking this would help. As I bent over I was so weak I just fell into the river. I'll bet some of the guys still chuckle when they think of that.

While I was forcing down a breakfast with lots of sand added to it I was given the details of the night before. It seems that my cousin Dale Thomas, for some reason—inner demons, low tolerance to alcohol, or whatever—decided to go on the rampage. The noise I had heard across the fire was Dale hitting Brad Rayfield in the back with a club, and then it was my turn. He said that my white socks were all that was visible when he was after me. He had large hillbilly bumps on his head where I had tried to put him to sleep.

As fate would have it Gene Shipton and Kenny Dixon happened by and put Dale out of commission. Since this book is not rated XXX, I will leave it to your imagination as to their method of restraint. I can laugh about it after so many years, but I vividly remember the feeling of sheer terror at being hunted by something or someone that means to harm you, and you are not only totally sightless but incapacitated to the point of being unable to defend yourself.

We were poster children for why young people, or anyone else for that matter, shouldn't mix intoxication with driving automobiles, shooting guns, or any activity which could prove to be potentially lethal.

Our senior year we decided to recapture our childhood with one last gathering in the woods. They say you can't go back, and this would soon be brought home to us in a poignant manner. It had been four years since our first camping expedition, and we were standing on the confusing and frightening threshold of adulthood.

Our campsite was located at Jerktail Landing on the Current River. There were five of us: Brad Rayfield, Brent Reary, Dale Thomas, John Counts, and me.

We set up camp on Friday afternoon, intending to have a great time. We had everything we needed to accomplish our mission. We had all the provisions necessary, such as alcohol, guns, food, and an abundance of misplaced energy.

Having set up camp and with plenty of daylight at our disposal, there was nothing left to do but slam down a few brews. (At this juncture, we had a healthy respect for whiskey.)

Soon we had a pretty good buzz going, and while roaming the river bank, we discovered a boat. A couple of the guys, after somehow disengaging the boat from its mooring, decided it would be fun to take a ride.

They did not concern themselves with legalities since the boat would be returned to its original location. Ah! The folly of youth!

I suppose in every group there is a father figure, and we had ours. His name was Brad Rayfield. He was my best friend, and was blessed with a greater sense of responsibility than the rest of us. He demanded that we leave the boat where it was since it did not belong to us.

A couple of the guys ignored Daddy and took a happy boat ride. Upon their return, however, things were not pleasant in paradise.

Our father figure friend was pissed. He had always been a hothead, but I believe the stress of passing from childhood to manhood took its toll, causing him to snap.

Suddenly, through the haze of the malt liquor, I realized he had a gun. It's a memory forever etched in my mind. We were seated around the campsite with an angry, red-faced teenager screaming and yelling

9

obscenities. He told us not to move. Hell! I couldn't have moved. I was petrified. It would not be the first nor the last time I would look down the barrel of a gun, and I can tell you it makes a lasting impression.

He was directing most of his rage at my cousin, Dale Thomas. As you may recall, he beat the hell out of everyone on our first camping trip. If Dale was frightened he didn't show it. He just sat there and smiled as if to say, "Shoot me, I don't care."

If this was fun I could live without it. It's like the blind cat said when he was making love with the porcupine: "I've enjoyed about as much of this as I can stand."

When things finally cooled down, John Counts and I made the decision to leave. That it was a nine-mile walk to town and that we were drunk on our ass and rapidly running out of daylight was of no consequence. We were getting the hell out of there.

Walking a few miles and sobering considerably, we began to question our decision, but we trudged on, and making it to the highway after a five-mile walk, we hitched a ride to town.

I showered, and being exhausted, was resting comfortably in bed when there was a knock at the door. It was John. He had borrowed his mother's car and wanted me to return with him to the campsite, intending to retrieve our camping gear.

Like a fool I agreed. I was at the wise old age of eighteen. Today, in a similar situation, I would laugh and return to the bliss and safety of my bed. But that would have been too easy, so instead we began the long, slow journey back to camp.

Cruising Ozark Mountain back roads in darkness one may become disoriented in a heartbeat, and that's exactly what happened to us. We found ourselves on the wrong road. After driving several miles we came upon some standing water, and as we attempted to turn around, the car sank to the wheels in mud.

What a nightmare. A short time before, I was snoozing in my bed after having walked for miles, only to find myself in the same situation once again. Was this really happening to me?

John elected to remain in the car. He couldn't bring himself to walk to town for the second time that night. As for me, I would return to my bed if I had to crawl on my hands and knees. I started walking.

I hadn't walked far when I realized this situation was unfamiliar to me. I was in the woods, blind, and totally alone. All sounds reaching my ears were instantly amplified. The sounds became a roar. I could hear things moving out there in "Natureland".

Keeping to the road was easy, for I had become quite skilled at utilizing my remaining senses, such as feeling the ground beneath my feet. What I couldn't control, however, was my imagination. Around 4 a.m., after a long, tiring, anxious walk, I finally made it home again!

Given the circumstances today, I could walk out of there in the middle of the night quite casually, but I was young, and therefore my mind was young. I have since learned that fear usually originates from one's imagination.

It's interesting to note that, five years later, my father would purchase a cabin on Current River. I would travel this road many times, and thirty-five years later I would once again find myself on the same road, blind, alone, disoriented, and frightened, but with one exception. The sun would be shining. (See chapter 8.)

During my youth someone came up with the idea of cave exploration. There were plenty of caves around to explore, so we chose one and strolled up to the entrance, then entered, not giving a second thought to hazards which might possibly lie ahead. Our cave exploration gear consisted of a flashlight. Very soon I would find that cave exploration would leave much to be desired. The first dose of reality would soon become apparent. Within seconds after entering the cave I was totally blind. The flashlight illuminated nothing for me, and adding to my dilemma, my fellow explorers, Randy Chilton and Brad Rayfield, were advancing as if we were in a race for our lives. Being one of the gang, I said nothing and tried to keep pace. I stumbled over rocks, stepped in holes, and many times my head would connect with the ceiling.

I am uncertain of the distance our journey took us into the dark bowels of the earth, a mile or more perhaps. There were times when we would crawl and at other times we would find ourselves in a large cavern. We had no markers or tether line to aid our escape from the cold darkness. Never mind that passages led in all directions. Somehow we always managed to return safely. When at last we would enter into sunlight once more, I always wanted to drop to my knees and thank God, but I said nothing. After all we were men, we were cave explorers.

I would be trembling from anxiety, scratched up as if I had tangled with a panther, with plenty of hillbilly bumps on my head.

I actually returned to the caves once more before my lesson was complete. After that when someone would mention caves I was nowhere to be found.

I must say we were getting creative. Someone came up with the idea of going coon hunting. I assure the politically correct animal lovers out there that the coons certainly had nothing to fear from us. It was a perfect plan. All young boys in the Ozark Mountains went "coon huntin'." This was our rite of passage. Our parents would certainly support this activity.

Of course we took guns and dogs along, and oh yes, did I mention whiskey? By this time we had learned our lessons well. We were respectful of what this "fire-water" could do to us—in other words, we sipped rather than gulped.

I tell the coon hunting story because once again I was thrust into darkness. I was not then, nor am I now, the type to be excluded from the action, and not only was I a city boy, but I was a blind city boy trying to be a country boy. We would sit around the fire and wait for the dogs to start running the coons. Then all hell would break loose. By this time we would be getting pretty loaded. Imagine, a bunch of teenagers running around the woods with guns, squalling dogs, and whiskey.

When the dogs would start chasing the coons we would take off after them. I would lag behind everyone trying to keep up. I would get slapped in the face by tree branches, run into tree trunks, stepped in holes, and fall over dead trees and rocks.

During one of these outings I stepped into a void while trying to keep up. I rolled end-over-end for what seemed like an eternity. I had stepped off a twenty-foot bank that was so steep you had to crawl rather than walk to make your way to the top again. As I was rolling down the bank, carrying with me leaves, rocks, and dead tree limbs, I was laughing as only a blind, drunk teenager could. All of my friends were laughing. The coons were laughing so hard they were falling out of the trees.

Finally, when they regained their composure, my so-called friends formed a chain and helped me ascend once more to the top of the bank. Needless to say, this was my last coon hunt.

Once again I was beat all to hell just because I wanted to fit in. Why does youth have to be wasted on the young?

Once upon a time in the mid-60s there was a roller rink at a place called Alley Spring, which was about six miles west of Eminence, Missouri, on Highway 106. Seldom did I miss being there on Friday nights. It was a good place for everyone to get together, and we had not at this point in time acquired total freedom. This would later arrive in the form of a driver's license.

We would skate most of the time at full speed as if we had lost our minds, darting in and out of the other skaters. I didn't know why, but I was starting to notice girls, and again my ego was about to lead me into trouble.

There were times when they would turn down the lights, and the boys and girls would put an arm around one another and gracefully skate around the rink. Yep, that's right, they turned down the lights. Now that should have been my first clue, but I was blinded by my ego as much as anything.

I don't know if Kay Ferguson asked me to skate with her or if I did the honors, but I can tell you that instead of saying, "No thank you, I can't see when the lights are down," I took her arm and away we went. If I would have had a blindfold over my eyes it would have been no different. I could see absolutely nothing. To hell with common sense, my ego was in control. I was out on that floor with my arm around a pretty girl, and I was one of the gang.

Then I was on my back. Voices and people were yelling. There were lots of brilliant colors and stars. I found myself stretched out on a bench. I had damned near been knocked unconscious.

Someone's head had found my eye. It's very sad, but it would be decades before I would begin to see the light.

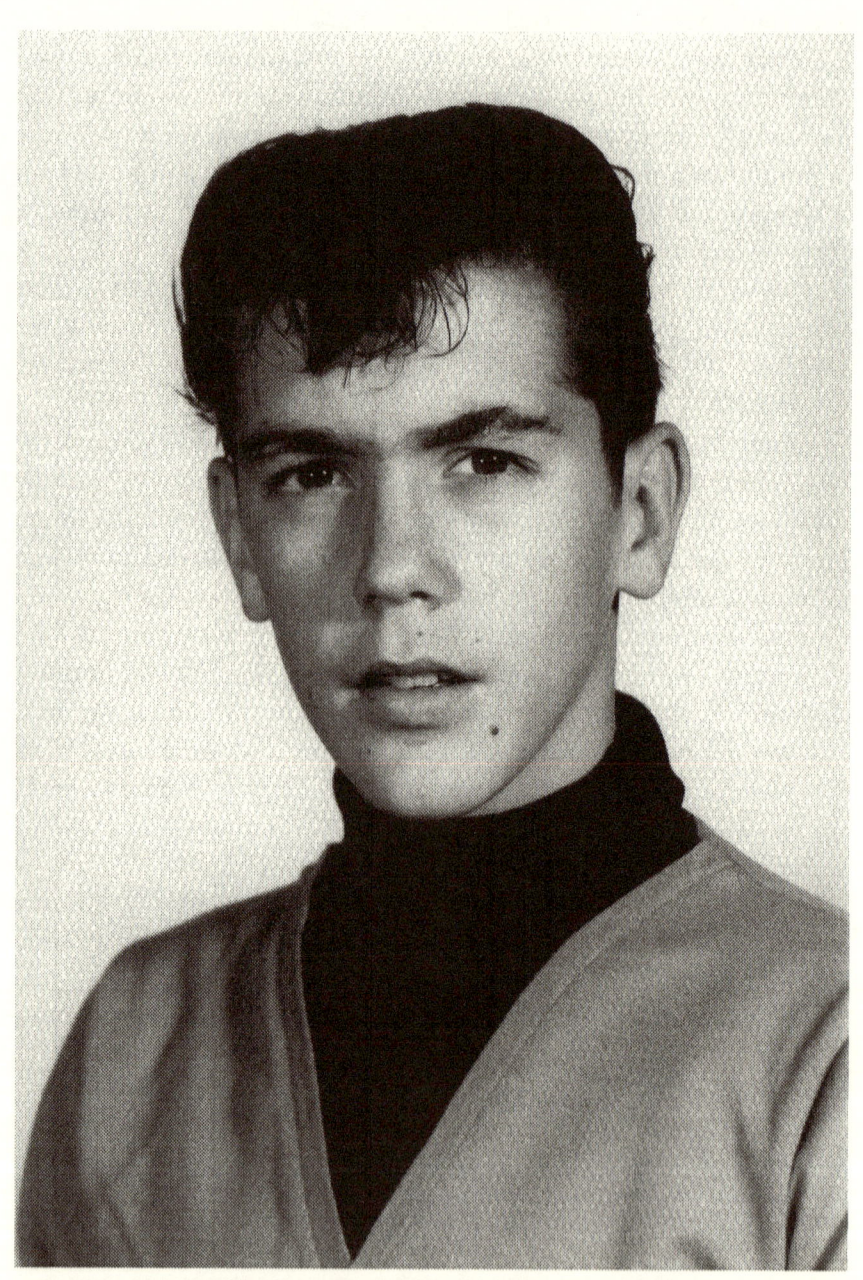

Freshman EHS (Eminence High School) 1964

Chapter 3
Driving Under the Influence of Blindness

In ancient times young Native American boys would take the scalp of their enemies to pass into manhood. In modern America, in order for a young boy to pass into manhood, he must first obtain his DRIVER'S LICENSE. This was especially true in the mid-60s, the time of hot rods and hot rod music. Every young man dreamed of cruising the streets of his hometown in his own wheels with his girl sitting next to him. I am sure this is still true today.

I began dreaming of motorcycles and cars when I was around fourteen. During the years that preceded the acquisition of my driver's license, not once did the fact that I had poor vision enter my hormone-ravaged mind.

The first time I took the driver's test I failed. This was not, however, due to my vision or lack of it. I blame my misfortune on a 1950 Chevy pickup truck that belonged to my great-grandmother and her husband. Need I say more? I was as nervous as a long-tailed cat in a room full of rocking chairs. I had studied for weeks and I was devastated, but in a few weeks I recovered soundly, having taken the test successfully in a more suitable automobile. To put it in teenager lingo of the time, "Wow, I got my wheels!"

Okay, I got my wheels, I'm "Mr. Cool," nothing can stop me now, right? Wrong. A few days after obtaining my so-called manhood I was chauffeuring my mother and grandmother to our home across the Jack's Fork River just north of Eminence. I was making a left turn at the entrance of the Riverside Motel, our place of residence at the time. Like a good little boy I had put my left turn signal on and had reduced my speed in order to execute the turn. My central vision was still with me. I scouted the highway ahead and there were no cars coming. My eyes went to the entrance and I began to make the turn. At this moment my grandmother, bless her soul, gasped and then yelled. My eyes returned to the highway just in time to see a car. Man, he was moving and he was heading straight for us. Our reaction was simultaneous. He took it to the shoulder of the road, and I whipped the wheel and took it back to my lane. He was giving me the horn while performing these life-saving maneuvers, and I couldn't blame him.

I remember my grandmother saying as I pulled into the motel, "We come very near gettin' killed right there." When I got out of the truck I could barely walk. Man, I was shaking like a whore in church. The thought of killing my mother and grandmother made me want to throw up.

What I didn't realize at the time was that, while I was trying to ignore it, my peripheral vision was deteriorating quite rapidly. That's the nature of my eye disease. First the peripheral vision goes, then you are left with central vision, and finally it too will abandon you.

A couple of years later someone told my mother, "Michael always looks both ways several times before he pulls out into traffic. That boy is one careful driver." I can assure you that if you were trying to drive a car while looking through a tube you would certainly scan the area before you made a move.

From that day on I was extremely cautious. During the daylight hours I would terrorize the highways of the Ozark Mountains. As I write this book it comes to mind that my grandmother never again rode in a vehicle while I was driving. What's up with that?

Carved on my tombstone should be the words, "Here lies a man that had to learn everything the hard way." Thus it has been throughout my time on this planet.

One would think, after the incident in which I very nearly killed myself along with my mother and grandmother, that I would have learned my lesson, but this time there was a woman involved, so what little sense I may have had at that time was completely dissolved.

I had been driving only a few weeks and during the daylight hours. I would not think of asking Mom and Dad for the car after the sun went down. Since my parents were fully aware of my vision problems and I would be driving their car, there was no way on God's green earth this was going to happen.

So it came to pass that my cousin Brenda Corbin was visiting from St. Louis. She had her own car, she was a couple of years older than I, and she was a fox. One night we were cruising the town, a couple of bored teenagers. We may have had a few beers. I thought, "This is my chance. Now I can find out if I can drive at night." Poor Brenda! She was young and fairly innocent. To this day, I'm sure she doesn't realize how much danger she was in. If she should read this book I may be in trouble.

I asked her if I could drive. She was reluctant at first. I told her that I had never driven at night. Again, my ego was working on me. I was supposed to be driving. I was with a pretty girl, and I was the male.

She finally relented, and I slid behind the wheel. I had been curious for months. I could see the white line but could hardly see the edge of the road. At that time there was open range in our area. If a cow wandered in front of this blind egomaniac it would become hamburger in short order. Brenda could sense that something was wrong. Duh, I was speeding along at 40 mph, and my face was only a foot from the windshield. I was doing okay until I met a car. Now we're talkin' serious blindness. I must have had an angel looking over my shoulder that felt sorry for me, because I was so stupid. Somehow we made it, and Brenda and I decided simultaneously that my night-driving lesson was over. I soon found a place to pull over, and as I was walking around the front of the car my legs could hardly carry me.

It would please me ever so much to tell you that I would never again take it upon myself to hazard the public roads while driving under the influence of blindness, and that I would never again endanger my life or the life of someone else, but as you will soon read in the following pages, this would not be the case.

The incident I will now describe is about having fun with blindness. I gradually learned over the years to have a sense of humor about my unfortunate situation. However, I was always ambivalent. Being a teenager, I was confused. Sometimes I could laugh and joke about it, and other times I wasn't in the mood to be reminded of it. Come to think of it, I am still that way. I can sense a person's intelligence. For instance, if some idiot says, "Man, I don't know how you can stand to be blind," my standard answer is, "I'd rather be blind than stupid." At the same time I can tell if someone is genuinely caring and sincere.

It's hard to imagine having fun with blindness, but it can be done. Living in a small town we had to make our own entertainment, and this was made easier when there was snow and ice on the ground. My buddy Rex Gates had an old '58 Chevy, and sometimes four or five of us would take it down to the ballpark after a good snow or ice storm. The ballpark was on the east side of Highway 19 just before you cross Jack's Fork River if you're going north.

It was an open field down there and we turned it loose. Since we are living in a police state, it wouldn't be wise to try that today, kids, for they would lock you up and throw away the key. Not to mention fine your ass thousands of dollars. We would take off until we reached a speed of 40 or 50 mph, the driver would jerk the wheel hard to the left or right, and then let the games begin.

I can still remember the roar of the engine and the tires spinning. There was snow and dirt flying everywhere, and we were laughing our hillbilly asses off. We would be turning doughnuts and still moving forward. I still can't believe that we didn't roll the car.

It was only natural that someone would think it quite entertaining to turn the blind boy loose and see what he could do in that ice-covered field. I was only too happy to oblige. After all, what could it hurt? I was in the middle of an open field.

I got behind the wheel and revved the engine. They had a plan. They would direct me in a straight line. In other words I would hold the wheel straight, and when we had reached the appropriate speed, they would give the signal, by which I mean they would yell "NOW," and I would jerk the wheel and we would spin like a top.

That was their plan, I had my own. I thought, "The joke's gonna be on you, boys." We started racing across the field and gaining speed.

Everyone was laughing and having a good ole' time! I noticed as we gained speed that it grew quiet in the car. Someone said, "Okay, get ready." By now I was grinning from ear to ear, because I knew we were running out of field and rapidly approaching the trees. Finally someone yelled "NOW!." I grinned wider and drove faster. This time there was fear in their voices. "They said, "NOW!" We were roaring across the field. They were no longer having fun, but I certainly was. I was laughing out loud. Everyone was yelling "NOW!" at the top of their lungs. "NOW!", had suddenly become a very popular word.

Finally, when they started grabbing for the wheel, I knew the time had come. We spun several circles. I had the gas pedal to the floorboard. The momentum was carrying us forward. I had no idea where we were. I expected to feel the car crash into the trees at any time. We stopped just a few yards at the edge of the field. The "Blind Fairy" had saved my ass.

We got out and stood around the car. I was still grinning, although I will admit that I cut it much closer than I wanted to. But I wasn't about to let them know that. They didn't know whether to laugh and pat me on the back or be pissed. I heard phrases like "McIntire, you son-of-bitch!" or "God-damn you, McIntire, I'm gonna kill your ass," but I knew they loved me and were proud of me, because they knew that I got 'em good. From that point on, when we turned doughnuts in the snow I was not, for some reason, invited to drive.

From 1966 until 1969 I rode a motorcycle. I had become quite skillful at scanning the roads with my limited vision while rolling at break-neck speeds over the winding roads of the Ozark Mountains. Consequently nothing extraordinary happened while riding the motorcycle, as long as it was parked before the sun had set. There were, however, several times when the blind Hells Angel wanna-be failed to return home before the sun had set. This was when things became quite extraordinary. Most of the time I would be in the company of one or more of my biker buddies, and I could simply follow their taillight and use it as a beacon to guide me. We would go to my house where I would park the bike and ride "bitch" with one of my friends.

It was a good plan, but things didn't always work out that way. Time would sometimes get away from me. I would be talking to a pretty tourist person of the opposite sex or just having too much fun with my friends, and before I knew it darkness would be upon me, and I would have to take myself and my motorcycle home.

It was during one of these momentous and dangerous excursions that my old friend David Beck had the misfortune to be my passenger. I've known Dave since he was in grade school. Dave loves to tell this story to anyone who will listen, and never mind that you may have heard the same story ten times before.

It was summer, and boys being boys, we were chasing tourist girls at Alley Spring Park, west of Eminence. I don't know what happened, but it was well after dark when we climbed on the bike and headed for home. Meeting a car was a nightmare. I just tried to avoid the car while keeping to the highway. Dave was about fourteen at this time and totally unaware of the life-threatening situation. The poor lad would soon become all too aware of the clear and present danger.

Again, the center line was all that guided me. Take this away and I was in trouble. There were sections of highway where the center line did not exist. I assume this was because the road had been repaired and not yet repainted. When this happened I would be thrown into a total and complete panic. Shortly, the white line would resume and I would breathe a sigh of relief.

Going into a curve I would instinctively lean down, hoping to gain a more precise view of the center line. Many years later Dave, while telling this story for the boys, would recall dramatically, "Man, every time he would lean down, the wind would damned near blow me off the bike. Hell, I thought he was lookin' at the motor or the tires or somethin'!"

The beauty of this story is when my young, innocent, fourteen-year-old buddy made the mistake of asking me, "What are you lookin' at down there?" As I write this I am laughing out loud. I would have loved to have seen the expression on his face when I yelled over my shoulder, "THE WHITE LINE."

The Blind Fairy helped us return safely to our destination, and for the remainder of the journey Dave kept his silence, and he also kept his fat hillbilly ass off the back of my motorcycle.

To this point I have shared with the reader frightening and sometimes humorous situations that only a blind man could find himself in while trying to operate a motor vehicle. The majority of these took place before graduation from high school. My ego as well as my idiocy, however, knew no bounds. Fortunately, by the time I had reached my late twenties I had begun to mature. As the years passed I slowly began to learn my limitations.

The summer of 1968 I attended my first semester at Southwest Missouri State University in Springfield. During my college years I seldom drove. Occasionally I would take my parents' car or my motorcycle to school for a week, returning to my home town the next weekend. Several years passed without incident.

In 1976 I bought my first vehicle with four wheels. I was proud of that van. I had purchased it with my own money.

I was living in Springfield. This time around most of my driving was done in the city. Man, I had to be on the ball, constantly alert. There were people and vehicles running in all directions. It was like an ant farm, and it's a hundred times more congested today.

I had owned my van but a few months when I was driving east on Elm Street just northwest of the SMSU campus. Naturally it was during daylight hours, but there was a heavy overcast. I approached a stop sign at the end of the block and brought the van to a stop as I had done hundreds of times before. Only this time it would be one of those life-changing moments.

Out of the corner of my eye I saw something. I glanced to the right, and I still have the look on that guy's face burned in my brain. He had most likely been running. He had arched his back to avoid being struck by the van. He was about four feet from where I sat. Our eyes locked for a second, and what I saw on his face was not anger or surprise but sheer terror. The poor guy looked like he was being chased by a grizzly bear. If he would have had a choice, I'll bet he would have taken a grizzly any day over a blind man driving a vehicle weighing thousands of pounds, unknowingly making him run for his life.

I missed that college student by no more than six inches. Needless to say, I didn't look back. I proceeded to get my hillbilly hippie ass out of there. I took that van home and parked it. Once again I was shaking like a whore in church. The next day I put a "For Sale" sign on that potentially lethal weapon, and never again would I drive in a metropolitan area.

Call it blind justice, but a few years later I found myself in the position of the horrified pedestrian. I was crossing a street near campus when I detected movement from the corner of my eye. Instinctively I leaped straight up, and as my hip struck the hood of the car, I rolled off the side of the instrument of destruction and landed on my feet unharmed. With trembling legs I kept walking.

I didn't look back, fearing I might gaze into the sardonic face of the college student I had nearly turned to road kill a few years earlier.

There were times, especially during the 70s, when my skills at being blind came into play. After a long night of indulging ourselves with various intoxicating substances, my friends and I would eventually decide that it might be prudent to take our tired body's home. There was not enough alcohol in the world to dull their senses to the point of asking me to drive. However, I remember on many occasions riding shotgun and wondering if I would make it to my home in one piece. Speed was not the problem because we rarely exceeded 30 or 40 mph.

This was a good thing because the driver would usually be slumped over the wheel trying to take a power nap while weaving from one lane to the other. It was easy for me to ascertain that we were no longer on the asphalt because of vibrations, sound, etc.

If I had a nickel for every time that, knowing my life was in danger, I had to scream at the top of my lungs, "God damn it, get back on the road," I would be a rich man today. Apparently this must have happened quite frequently, for many people of Shannon County will not soon forget the night they returned safely to their home, due in part to the acute senses and stark terror of a blind man.

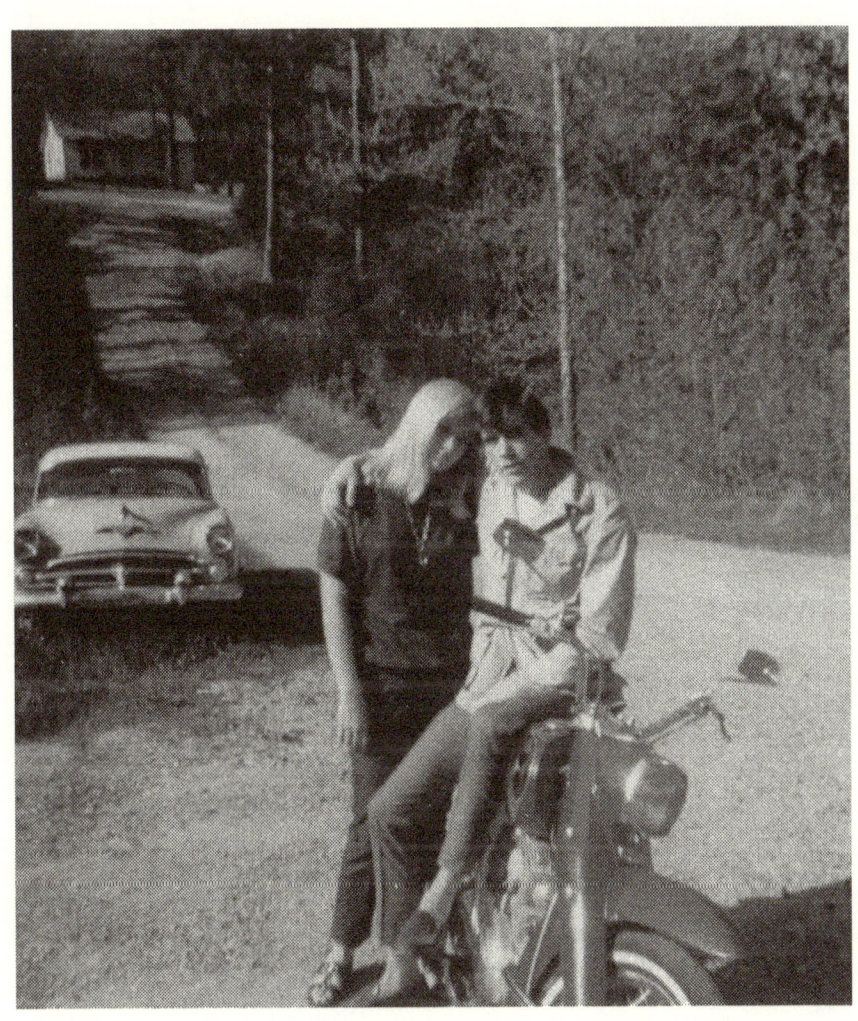

Michael and Jeanie McCallister, 1968

Chapter 4
Sir! Could I See Some Identification?

It was around 1977 that I was informed by the great state of Missouri that by law I had to renew my driver's license. At this time I was driving a white '55 Chevy previously owned by Phil Titus. The '55 was a legend in our home town. It was the champion of many drag races across the Jack's Fork River Bridge and at "The Graveyard Stretch" south of town. Man, that thing would run, but I was just a spaced out hippie cruising around with my dog. Even though I was limited to daylight driving, I still would not have wanted to forfeit this privilege.

Needless to say, I was apprehensive about taking the test again. Missouri had come up with a new test for side vision. It didn't look good. By now I was declared "legally blind." Oh God, it felt so good to finally be declared legal. I used to be illegally blind; now I'm a card-carrying cool, blind cat.

So anyway I showed up at the court house at the appointed hour on the appointed day. I knew I was in trouble when I stepped through the door. It was as dark as a witch's hat. I followed the highway patrolman to the machine where I was to take the eye exam. All I had to do was follow the sound of those big leather Nazi boots he was wearing.

He told me to have a seat. Yeah, right, like I knew where the seat was, but as usual I faked it. I started walking, having absolutely no idea where I was going. I took about three steps and immediately kicked a metal trash can across the room. I can still hear the roar of that trash can as it rolled and tumbled across the hard floor. I listened to each echo with a heavy heart, for I knew that no one in their right mind would give me a driver's license. All was lost.

There was no way in hell that I was going after that can because I knew that I would never find my way back.

To my surprise the officer simply said, "It's down at this end." I took the test knowing with certainty that I was wasting the State's time as well as my own.

After that little incident I would have expected to be spread-eagled against the wall and searched for drugs.

Weeks went by and I was making plans to sell my car, for I knew that I would have no need of it. Then one day an envelope addressed to yours truly arrived from the state. I very nearly threw it in the trash, for I knew the outcome. Reluctantly I opened it and for a short moment I thought I was visually impaired, for there looking back at me was myself, triumphant grin and all.

The picture did me justice. I had shoulder-length hair at the time and was probably stoned. I just stood and stared. There it was, my DRIVER'S LICENSE. I was good to go for a few more exciting years. The Blind Fairy was still in my corner.

For the next couple of years I was pretty mellow. I cruised around town in my '55 Chevy. Sometimes, just for a cheap thrill, I would get on it. There was still something special about the roar of the engine, the smell of burning rubber, and being thrown back in the seat while going through the gears.

In 1979 Roger Sanders and I set out across the country in the Chevy. By this time my vision had deteriorated further. I knew it was time for this blind boy to remove himself from the driver's seat. I had learned to drive on the roads around my home town, so yeah, I could almost do it with my eyes closed, but I had no desire to test my luck at cross-country driving. It had been a great adventure and I had lived through it, but I knew that if I entered that cave-like courthouse to take my vision test to obtain a driver's license for the third time, I would have the aid of a white cane or a guide dog. Also, presented with this evidence it's quite possible that the man with the big black leather Nazi boots just might get wise to me.

A person of reasonable intelligence would think that a blind man riding shotgun where he belongs, legally or otherwise, would be quite safe from confrontation with the law. That is, laws pertaining to the operation of a motor vehicle. Right? WRONG!

If we are stopped at night it's always the same routine. "Sir, would you please remove your sunglasses?" I now look respectable but it doesn't matter. They just assume that I must be chemically challenged. Next they wish to see my DRIVER'S LICENSE. Someone's playing a cruel joke. Maybe the word got out about the metal trash can. It is taken for granted that American citizens own two things. That would be a dog and a driver's license.

I was in a vehicle which was detained by the highway patrol as recently as 2003. The patrolman, a child of about twenty-three years of age, asked for my license. Having gone through this for the last four decades, I got creative. I said in a deep, cool voice from behind my shades, "Son, the good citizens of the great state of Missouri would not take kindly to it if I were to attempt the operation of a motor vehicle on the public roads and highways. I couldn't see him, but I could visualize the "deer in the headlights" look. My friend, Gary Alcorn, chuckled. Finally, after testing his sense of humor to the limit, I showed him my Missouri I.D.

Eventually I obtained a Missouri I.D. complete with picture, although it says "female." You think maybe the old redneck working at Springfield City Hall was trying to tell me he didn't like my long hair? Yeah, I still had my driver's license, but have you ever tried to convince a cop you are legally blind while he is standing there holding your license in his hand?

The first time this happened to me I was attending an Ozark Mountain Daredevils concert in Springfield around 1977. By this time the audience consisted mostly of Mom, Dad, and the kids. I shouldn't have been there and I knew it. I was roaming around with hair down to my ass, wearing shades, and I couldn't see shit, but what the hell, I had free tickets.

Suddenly a cop came up to me and said, "Come with me." They took me into a room, and I was surrounded by no less than fifteen cops. By this time I was a veteran, and I knew I was clean, so I let them have it. I demanded to know what this was about. Finally one of them said, "Well, I don't know, something about you is just not right." Well, you can imagine how that set me off.

After that I had them chasing their tails. I didn't scream or yell like they do on the television show *Cops*, but when the interrogation concluded; they were more than happy to send me on my way.

As usual, they asked for my operator's license. I gave it to them. Then amazingly they wanted to know why I was running into things. I told them I was legally blind, and one of the more intelligent officers asked how it was that I could have a driver's license if I was legally blind. I said, "I'm from a small town. You know how it is. Go ahead, give them a call." If they would have called my bluff I would have had a lot of explaining to do.

They held me for an hour or so before my freedom was granted. That was my wake-up call. I threw my driver's license in a drawer, and from then on the law could gaze upon my Missouri I.D. I hope they consider Michael McIntire to be one very ugly female.

I couldn't count the number of times during my life the law wanted to see my driver's license. I will highlight the stories most memorable to me.

In 1987 I had just returned from Hawaii and was cruising around town with my cousin Mark Williams. We were crossing the Jack's Fork Bridge when we met a state trooper coming from the opposite direction. Mark said, "If he turns around hang on." In 1987 I could still see a little in the daylight, and when I looked back I could see the trooper turning around. Mark was already getting the hell out of Dodge. He turned left at the end of the bridge on what is now called Tom Akers Drive. How ironic, a road named after the local astronaut and my cousin and myself are about to play "Dukes of Hazard" on it.

At that time it was a gravel road, and within seconds we were running 50 or 60 mph. I thought I was dreaming. I couldn't believe I was in this situation. The first curve we came to was at the Steel Bridge Hole. We took the curve sliding sideways. If another car had been coming from the opposite direction I am sure there would have been a head-on collision.

Suddenly there was a loud roar, and the car started bouncing up and down. I knew it was more than a blown tire. We immediately skidded to a complete stop.

Before I knew it Mark was out and running. I was in shock. I sat there for a second and then it hit me. The trooper was right behind us, and I'd better get my hippie hillbilly ass out of there. As I stepped from the car I could see Mark splitting the brush. He was making his way through a briar patch. I was thirty-seven years old, and it took about a second to come to the conclusion that I would sooner spend time in jail than get scratched to pieces in a briar patch.

Visualize this. Mark is a big guy. I would guess his weight around three hundred pounds. Remember those African movies when the elephant is crashing through the jungle?

I started walking back to town, and guess what? I could here a car headed my way, and he was not out for a leisurely drive. My plan was to be out of sight of Mark's car by the time the cop reached my position, but this was not to be. A few seconds later and I would have made it.

The cop stopped beside me, and I walked to his car with a big smile on my face. The guy was all of twenty-four. I was only thirty-seven, but I felt like grandpa.

He asked if I had seen a car go speeding by. "No sir," I said. One thing you don't do in the hills is rat on people, especially your relatives. I told him I was just walking to town. I knew he couldn't be that stupid. He wasn't.

We returned to Mark's car and wouldn't ya know it, he wished to see my operator's license. I got out my Missouri I.D. He wanted to know if I was driving that car. By now I was beginning to lose patience. I had been there, done that, and have the t-shirt. I had told him that I was legally blind, but as I said this I was looking into his eyes because it was daylight and I could still see through the tunnel. I said, "If you don't believe me, ask them."

By now half the town had arrived. They must have seen the big chase scene.

"This is a popular place," he said.

"Yeah, around here you take your excitement where you find it," I said. "Go ahead. Ask them. They'll tell you I'm blind. Hell, I'm related to half of them."

By now I was thoroughly enjoying myself. People were slowly driving by the scene. The citizens knew everything and the policeman knew nothing. They were grinning like a butcher's dog, for they were aware that Mark had run and left me to explain things to the law.

The patrolman was a cool guy. He shrugged and said, "It doesn't matter, I'll get him in a few days." He knew Mark and I believe his instincts told him that I was telling the truth.

I was driven back to town by one of the locals, Luke Stewart. He took much delight in telling me why the chase ended so abruptly.

It seems that the rear axle along with the rear wheels became disengaged from the car. It reminded me of a sled on gravel after running out of snow.

A few days later about twenty or thirty of us were standing around shootin' the breeze at the maintenance shed when our buddy the patrolman pulled up in his cruiser. We said our goodbyes to Mark and wished him well and told him that we hoped to see him soon. (The maintenance shed is just inside the city limits of Eminence. It was a local gathering place. The locals tell me that gatherings such as this are no longer tolerated. In my travels I found that this is common throughout the country. Sound familiar? At the risk of becoming political, it is my opinion that we have fewer rights and freedoms in this country today than could be enjoyed yesterday.)

To this day I have no idea what Mark's punishment was. I have been meaning to ask him for sixteen years. They say he is in Florida. I wonder if he has lasting scars from the briar patch.

As I've said before, my life has been one crazy scene after another. I don't know how much of this can be attributed to my poor eyesight. Maybe it was my adventurous spirit. I am inclined to believe that both of these played a part.

There are many "May I see your identification, please" stories I could relay to you, but I will bring this chapter to a conclusion by telling you the story of my old friend Bill Fulks. It was around 1985 and Bill and I were roommates in Springfield, Missouri.

I was playing music at a bar called Lindburg's, on Commercial at Campbell. Bill was there with his truck and he was to give me a lift home. I had been drinking and playing guitar for about six hours, so I was feeling no pain. We loaded the equipment in his truck and everything went fine. I can sense when someone is too drunk to drive, and Bill seemed okay. Those of you who have had the extraordinary experience of knowing our friend Bill will certainly agree with me when I tell you that Bill's guitar is not always in tune.

We hadn't driven a block when I knew I was in trouble. I couldn't understand how anyone could get that drunk so quickly. He didn't know where he was or what he was doing. At times he was completely on the wrong side of the street. I remember yelling at him, "What the hell are you doing?" This was not the country. We were in the city, and in the big city they didn't take you home to Mommy so she could tuck you in. They took your ass to jail.

We were approaching an intersection, and I could plainly see the red traffic light. As I write this book I am capable of seeing traffic lights, street lights, car headlights, etc. I was certain that Bill would stop at the intersection. Well, he drove right through it. By this time I had had enough. I said, "You idiot, you'd better hope there's not a cop around here." As I said this I was turning to look behind us and sure enough, I saw the flashing lights. I thought, "Well Mac, here we go again."

The cop pulled us over and requested that Bill step out of the car. Thoroughly disgusted, I sat and listened as Bill made damned sure that he would not be driving for some time.

If it hadn't been so late and I hadn't been so tired it would have been hilarious. Bill could barely stand, so how was he to walk a straight line? I knew we were in trouble when Bill was going through the alphabet, struggling to pronounce the letters to "j" and then slurring his words and trailing off into space.

My first thought was, "How the hell am I going to get home?" As I sat there I devised a plan. I had been here many times and I thought, "If you sons of bitches leave me here without a ride and as blind as a bat, being a musician I know the media, and I promise you that we will be on the evening news tomorrow."

Finally, the cop came around the car to visit yours truly. I knew what was coming but to my surprise, he didn't ask for my I.D. Instead, he asked me to touch my fingers to my nose. I wish everything in life was that easy! I was going to milk this for all it was worth. When he asked me to recite the alphabet I did so with such speed and enunciation that I'll bet he's never heard a recitation of the ABCs done in such a manner. I was wound tighter than an eight-day clock. Had I not spent the entire evening playing the fire out of an electric guitar? My irritation had turned to amusement.

I couldn't understand why they didn't ask for my driver's license. Finally, after about thirty minutes of the same old bullshit that I had gone through for years, Mr. Policeman says, "Okay, you can drive the truck home." Man, I couldn't believe my ears, a blind man had passed the sobriety test and they were going to be so sweet as to let him drive the god damned truck home. Gee thanks guys, I could never thank you enough.

First the state allows me to obtain two driver's license in my lifetime and now, years later, I have passed a sobriety test and they are going to let my hippie hillbilly blind ass drive home.

I was ready for them. I had my very own MISSOURI I.D. We went through the usual routine. I had to convince them that I was blind. The cop said, "Why didn't you tell me you were blind?" This was the moment I had been waiting for. I felt all warm inside. "You didn't ask," I said with more satisfaction than I could convey to you.

By this time the paddy wagon had arrived. They were going to give my psychotic buddy a free ride and room and board for the night. They knew I was blind, and I was interested to see what my fate would be. I could overhear their conversation, and they had come up with a plan. I was to ride in the paddy wagon with the driver. Thank God. I might have killed Bill if I had been forced to ride in the back with him. The truck would be sent for later. I smiled to myself. Once again I felt that warm feeling inside, for I knew that I was about to experience something that I had never experienced before nor would I ever experience again.

The cops said, "Okay, let's go." We were all going to take a happy little ride on the jolly wagon. I said, "Wait a minute, what about my band equipment?" Bill was driving an open-bed pickup, and it was loaded with speakers, microphone stands, amplifiers, guitars, etc. It's times like this I wish I could see. I'll bet I would have seen that deer-in-the-headlights look again.

Try to picture this. Bill sitting in the paddy wagon probably not knowing where he is, and the cops are loading Michael McIntire's band equipment right in next to him. My music had finally been arrested. I was standing there savoring every second of this. That was my precious moment. It was well worth the trouble I had gone through.

As if the night had not been crazy enough, the guy driving us home in the paddy wagon for some reason felt the need to impress me. He wanted me to know that he was cool too. He told of his drug dealing days. He was still trying to impress me with his stories as the cops were unloading the band equipment into my house. For some reason I wasn't listening.

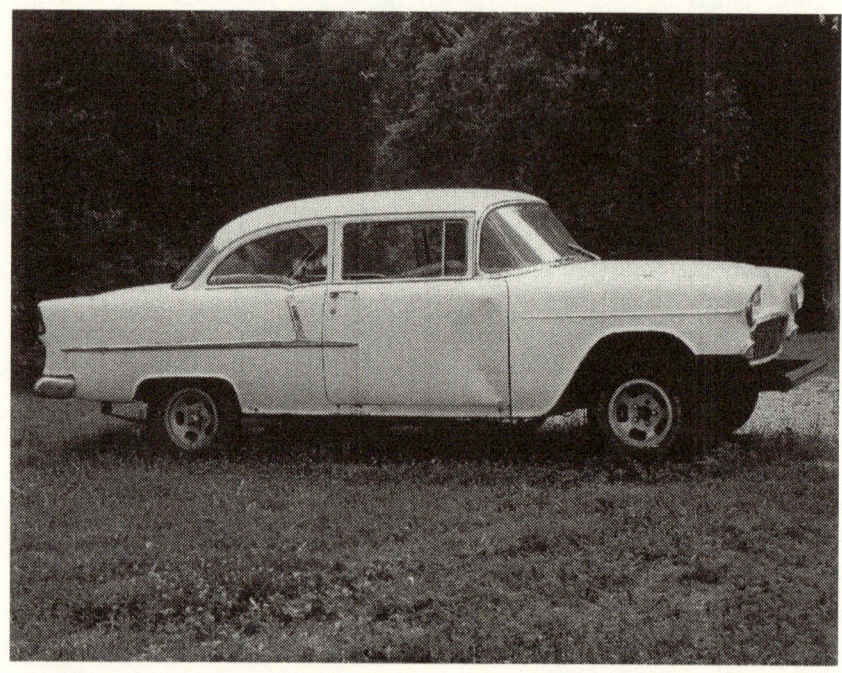

Having been a legend, in my hometown of Eminence, Missouri, this 55 Chevy was my pride and joy. In 1979, while touring the country pick'n and grin'n, Roger Sanders and myself, found ourselves in Springfield, Missouri, where we saw a beautiful blonde, hitching a ride. We moved in for the kill, but unfortunately, the guy in front of us, had the same idea.

The pavement was wet, and when he cut in front of us, Roger hit the brakes, causing the Chevy to go into a spin.

At the time, I had limited vision, but I could see the other car's rear bumper as it grew closer. My concern was for my car, rather than myself.

I guess the Blind Fairy wasn't ready for my life to end because of raging hormones, but she left a dent in my dream car, as something to be taken from the experience.

Chapter 5
Bottomless Pit

During the '60s and '70s there was a black blues club called BeBop's located just outside the city limits of Springfield. 1974 was a memorable year for me because, for the first time in my life, I was bitten by the love bug. Her name was Roxanne Kinsey.

One night we were all out at BeBop's having a good time. As usual there was a large crowd. The place was packed and there were probably a hundred people milling around outside the club.

On this particular night I was so messed up I could hardly walk. There was a light fixture on the wall of the building. I could see a few people standing under the light. One of them happened to be Roxanne, so I staggered in her direction. She turned toward me and then I found myself falling through black space.

It was like a dream. I was totally relaxed. I was resigned to my fate. Then came a huge crash. It was McIntire's limp body coming to rest upon tin cans and broken bottles.

It seems that I had fallen off an old wooden bridge that lay across a huge ditch that had been used as a dump for many years. They had to carry me out of there. For some reason I found humor in this. I was laughing my hippie hillbilly ass off. I came out of it without a scratch. Thank God, I was sufficiently anesthetized.

In 1980 I lived in Eminence with the mother of my twin daughters, Bebe Bryant, and her son Jeremiah. My daughters, Dillan and Dane, were still but a twinkle in their daddy's eye.

We lived on what is called School-House Hill, inside the city limits. One night after a disagreement with Bebe, I decided to take myself downtown.

I started walking. I wasn't worried because I had been walking alone at night for years. (This was before I had the good sense to use a cane.) It had always been easy for me to tell when I had stepped from the pavement onto the shoulder.

I reached the bottom of the hill near the post office. All of a sudden I was falling through that black void again. It was a concrete drainage ditch, the depth of which was at least six feet. It was right next to the pavement, so there was no warning. I just stepped into it. I can tell you that it scared me silly—not only was I no longer angry but I couldn't recall what had made me angry in the first place.

I wasn't hurt, but I was shaking like a leaf on a tree. The Blind Fairy was looking after me.

They tell me the ditch is still there, so if you walk that stretch of road at night, be you blind or blind drunk I suggest not only that you use a cane but that you be very attentive.

In 1985 I found myself at a party in Springfield. A few of my good buddies from "Booger County" were there. (Booger County is the local nickname for Shannon County.) If my memory serves me well, they were Greg Colyott, Red Deatherage, Tom Elmore, and Robby Nash. We were just milling around, shootin' the shit, which seems to be the most popular thing to do at a party. As one might expect, there was alcohol and other party treats.

It was early and I was far from catching a good buzz. Some of the guys were gathering at the back porch, so yours truly decided to join them. As I walked through the door I stepped to the left to allow the storm door to close. Suddenly I was falling through space. Words cannot describe the horrible experience. It's similar to an automobile wreck. One moment all is well, and then for no apparent reason your life could be brought to an end. Time slows down. As you are falling through the black void, you are wondering how far you will fall and what will greet you when you arrive at your destination. I can assure you that, had I been intoxicated, my journey would not have been so frightening. As it was I could already hear the ambulance and I was still falling through space.

After falling for what seemed like forever I finally crashed to the bottom. I could feel wire and steel. There was a big crash, and in the distance I could hear my buddies yelling. With much concern they gathered around me. They extracted my poor shocked body from the tangled mess.

There was much yelling and people shuffling around. As I took inventory of myself I realized that I had come through this ordeal without a scratch. The Blind Fairy had not forsaken me.

It seems I had stepped onto a concrete landing about five feet by four feet. There were no guard rails of any kind. If that were to happen to me today, it would be litigation city.

I had fallen into a basement stairwell beneath the porch. My fall was broken by several bicycles. This was better than landing on the concrete floor, but not much.

In 1999 I had a great idea. I would go to a nutritionist and get healthy. I made an appointment at a clinic next door to St. John's Hospital in Springfield. On the day of my appointment I was sitting in the waiting room with perfectly healthy people who were, like me, seeking nutritional advice.

I had been waiting for what seemed like an eternity. I had been to the restroom once and felt the need to return. The door to the restroom was approximately 12 feet from my seat. I was using my cane and had successfully navigated this distance before and saw no reason why this could not be done a second time. I had done my business and was returning to my seat when, to my complete and utter horror, I stepped into a bottomless pit.

Man, I freaked. My first thought was that I had stepped into an elevator shaft. It was like nightmares that I've had in the past. You know the abyss! You just keep falling and falling, only this was not a dream. It was real.

Out of pure desperation I yelled like they do in the movies. Talk about dramatic.

I rolled head-over-heels. At one point during my descent I saw a beautiful white light. I had struck my head on a concrete wall which lined the stairwell.

Imagine a six-foot two-inch man weighing 200 pounds doing cartwheels down a flight of stairs yelling his ass off in a nice, quiet, and very polite hospital. I like attention, but I can certainly think of better ways of getting it.

When the tumbling finally stopped I was sprawled flat of my back, about half-way down twenty-three steps. My head was at the lower end of the steps and my feet were above me. I was spread out like dinner on the ground.

My body was numb from head to toe. I thought, "This is it. You've really done it this time. I hope they have an extra hospital bed for you, Mac, 'cause you're busted all to hell." I figured the Blind Fairy had finally turned her back on me.

The next thing I knew there were nurses all around me. If you're gonna break your neck, what better place than a hospital? I wanted to check myself out, but they wouldn't let me move a muscle. They put a neck brace on me and threw my weak and shaking body on a stretcher faster than you can say "blind hippie hillbilly."

I was carried next door in an ambulance—can you believe that?—where I was given a thorough examination. I was scratched up a little but that was all. My Blind Fairy was still with me.

At the place where I had fallen there were no guard rails. It was just a hole in the middle of the floor. That could be dangerous for anyone.

In the weeks following the accident I received many calls from the hospital concerning my state of health. I would hope their concern was genuine; however, the word "litigation" comes to mind.

In the early '90s Debbie Hediger and I had just successfully completed a gig in Hot Springs, Arkansas. Not being ready to call it a night, we dropped by a local club to listen to the band. I was invited to sit in. The band was very good so I accepted. I strapped in and things were going great. The club was huge, and it was packed with around three hundred patrons. The dance floor was full and yours truly was rockin', as was the band.

The stage was large and there were about seven of us jamming. I remember being lost in the music, which is nothing uncommon for me.

When facing the audience, I was on the right side of the stage. While blissfully floating through musical la-la land, I must have unknowingly stepped to the right. Once again I had stepped into the void.

I had no idea how high the stage was from the dance floor, but this time I would not have time to panic, for my fall would be a short one. The height of the stage was only eight inches, just enough to make my heart stop and take my breath away.

Somehow I managed to stay on my feet and I didn't miss a beat. If anyone noticed my demise, it wasn't mentioned. I am speaking of the general public of course. Debbie watched my every move, but there was nothing she could have done to help me.

Over the years I have recalled the Hot Springs incident many times, and I am forever grateful that the stage was not five or six feet from the main floor as many are.

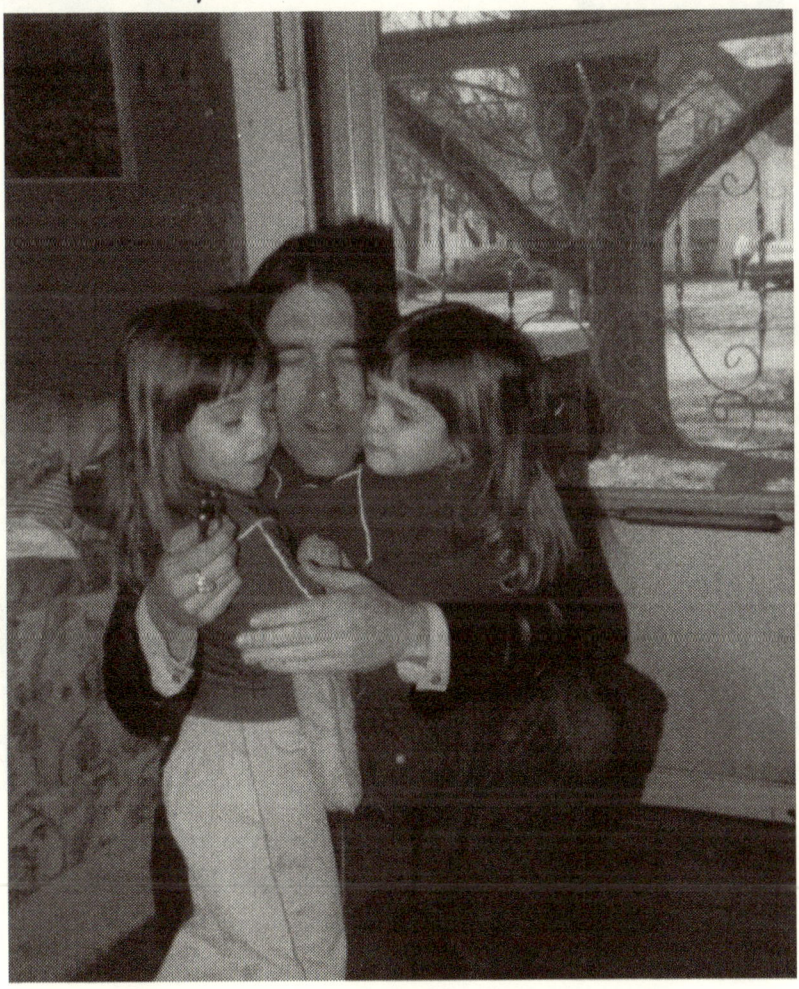

Michael and twin daughters, Dillan and Dane

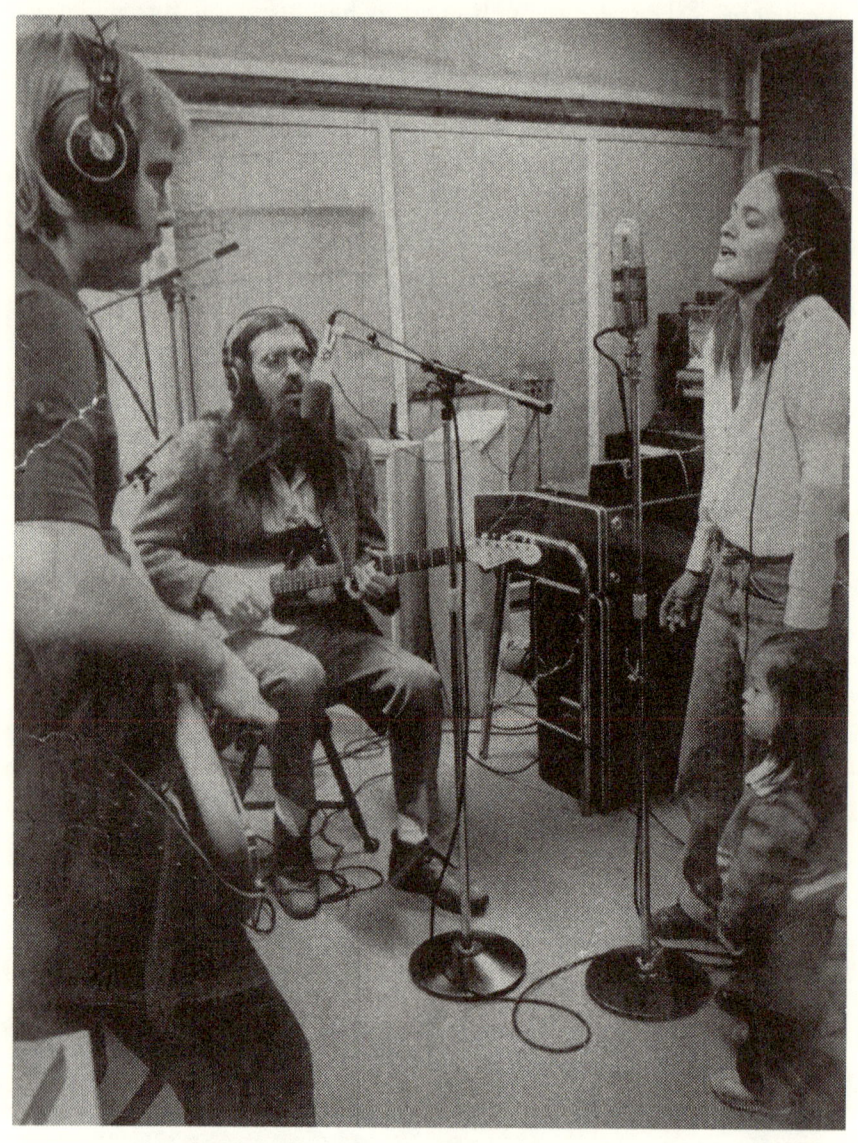

Michael and Bebe Bryant (Mother of Twins)
during the recording session of the album Runn'in Wild.

Chapter 6
Are You Laughing at Me?

It took many years but I finally learned to laugh at myself, and in retrospect I have found humor and entertainment in my particular situation. I am sure that some blind people will find this book offensive. To those poor, pitiful people I say, "Laugh and the world laughs with you, cry and you cry alone." I have much more to say to these idiots, but I promised my dear mother that I would refrain from using the "F" word in this book.

The years have taught me to accept my situation, and also to have fun with it. I have also learned—the hard way—not to take myself too seriously.

Here is a good example of my frame of mind as an eighteen year old. It was my senior year, and we were having band practice at Robert Deel's house. For those of you who are interested, the band was called The Vibrations.

On this particular night Danny Deatherage, a classmate, was hanging out with us.

We constantly teased and joked around as young people do. During practice Danny had mentioned my poor vision several times in jest. These days when this happens, as it frequently does, I just come back with something like, "I'd rather be blind than stupid," then everyone has a good laugh and moves on.

My hormones must have been in overdrive that night or maybe I was experiencing an extra dose of insecurity, for every time he made fun of my lack of vision it stung like a wasp. I realize now that it was just a symptom of those crazy years when we are passing from childhood to adulthood.

It was never my nature to be violent, but something snapped within me. I un-strapped my guitar and said to Danny, "Come on outside and I'll show you what a blind guy can do."

I assumed he was following me, but when I got outside and turned around he was not there. This only served to further infuriate me. I started screaming obscenities and begging him to come out. In my mind I was fixin' to climb him like a tree.

When I saw that he wasn't coming out I went in and strapped on my guitar, and we resumed playing music. Later I felt shame for what I had done, but the incident was never mentioned again, and as I recall, there were no more blind jokes.

Danny is a good guy and we speak from time to time. The Blind Fairy may have been watching over me that night because, for all I know, Danny could have thoroughly kicked my blind hippie hillbilly ass.

Hundreds of crazy things have happened to me through the years. My ego must be solid, for it has certainly taken a beating. During a road trip with a band in the mid-'70s we stopped at a filling station, and as I followed my friends inside, the door wouldn't open. I stood there and pulled on it but to no avail. I jerked and pulled, but it just wouldn't budge. I couldn't figure out what was wrong with the damned thing.

I finally looked up to see everyone in the building staring at me. Taking another look, I saw that the door was propped open, and I had been beside it pulling on the handle. There was only one thing I could do. I smiled and shook my head. After all, it was just another day in the life of a blind man.

A similar incident took place at college. I was to meet some friends at the library. As I entered the building, I happened to see my friends sitting around a table. I immediately began walking toward them.

There was a loud bang as I was suddenly smashed in the face and stopped in my tracks. "What the hell is going on?" I thought.

I had walked into a plate glass window. I was indeed getting an education, but it would not come from a book.

Around 1986 I was on the road with a band. We were in Cheyenne, Wyoming, and I had told the band leader what he and his wife could do with their poor excuse for a country band. I was a thousand miles from home with a guitar, amplifier, suitcase, and poor vision.

Sure, I was apprehensive, but I would have crawled home rather than remain in that abusive situation.

I flew from Cheyenne to Denver in a small prop job with no problem. Stapleton Airport was a different story. There were thousands of people running in every direction. I had to haul ass because my plane was at the other end of the airport. It would soon be leaving without me, and I wasn't about to let that happen.

As I was briskly walking along I looked to my right and could see the silhouettes of people, and they were just standing there moving at the same speed as I was. It came to me that I should hitch a ride on this moving sidewalk. I could not only save energy but could possibly save the life of some little old lady who might happen to find herself in my path.

As it happened I spotted one of those moving sidewalks directly ahead. When my feet stepped upon the moving sidewalk I immediately knew something was terribly wrong. I had planned to just stand there, but I found myself jogging in place. I looked up and people were on the moving sidewalk and headed straight for me. You can imagine how this was frying my brain. My ride on the moving sidewalk was a short one, lasting about three seconds. How I managed to stay on my feet I will never know. It finally dawned on me to just stand there and let the moving sidewalk take me in the direction from which I had come.

As I collected myself I looked about me. I had become a point of interest to hundreds of people.

Not one person laughed at my crazy dance on the moving sidewalk. On the contrary, I saw fear and concern in their eyes. Seeing a musician with hair down to his ass, they probably thought I was stoned out of my mind on drugs.

I took from that experience an important lesson. When you are far from home, make certain you are with people whom you can trust and rely upon. Especially if you are blind! I have yet to repeat this mistake.

In the late '90s Barbara Hoskin and I were performing at an AmVet's club north of Springfield, Missouri. While on break I was led to the restroom door. As is my custom I made my presence known upon entering the room by asking, "Is anyone in here?" Logic would dictate that if I hear no response I could consider myself to be alone.

Having properly announced myself, and soliciting no response, I stepped forward and began to make preparations to take care of business. The zipper was down, and all necessary equipment was made ready.

As I reached the facility, I realized to my horror and utter astonishment that I was not alone. The urinal was occupied.

What a position to be in. I damned near suffered cardiac arrest. I don't embarrass easily, but this situation certainly got the job done.

I was beside myself. Apologizing about twenty times, I made certain the guy knew I couldn't see. He got the hell out of the way and didn't utter a sound. His silence was most disturbing.

When we resumed the show, I couldn't play guitar, sing, or remember the lyric. A few songs into the set, I finally collected myself. At the end of the set—guess what?—I had to visit the little boy's room again.

This time as I opened the door I yelled at the top of my lungs, for once bitten, twice shy, and that's putting it mildly.

There was no response so I slowly made my way forward, and that's when I heard it. I was not alone.

There was a shuffling sound as someone moved to my left, from directly in front of me. He said, "I'm gettin' out of your way this time."

If I live to be a thousand years of age, I'll never understand people. I did everything I could to make certain he was aware of my blindness. I wore the complete costume, consisting of sunglasses and cane. I went so far as to ask if he was there. This reaffirms my belief that we can take nothing for granted—something blind people are never allowed to forget.

Around the year 2000 I was on the road playing music, and my partner at the time, Barbara Hoskin, had a daughter, Jamie, who was to be married in Las Vegas. I hadn't been there since 1969. It was not my kind of place then, and it damned sure wasn't my kind of place in the year 2000.

We were walking single file through the casino to the chapel where the wedding was to take place. There were thousands of people. My senses were assaulted from every direction. Little bells and whistles going off at all times, not to mention people yelling and walking as fast as their feet would carry them in every direction. They walk like they drive, full speed ahead. It reminded me of an international airport, but more chaotic. People were packed like sardines.

We were making our way through this madness in single file with Barbara and me in the lead. Barbara's parents, Al and Anne Johnson, were behind us.

These days, when in public places, I wear my dark glasses and white cane so people will get the idea that I'm blind and get the hell out of my way. One would think this would be sufficient, but believe me when I tell you that it isn't. I would love to have a cane with an electric jolt, such as a cattle prod, but I'm not sure even that would help.

After having walked what seems to be about two miles of trying to make our way through the crowded casino, I was rapidly losing patience. I was holding my cane in front of me and swinging it from side to side. Barbara later told me that some people were jumping over the cane trying to avoid possible injury from a blind man on the loose.

It was during this time that I felt someone's feet get tangled in my cane. Instantly I pulled the cane toward me, but this action was in vain. I heard the unmistakable slap of flesh hitting the hard surface of the floor.

I remember thinking to myself, "Man, you've done it now, McIntire. You're fix' to get your lights punched out." Not only did I not stop, but I picked up the pace. From behind me I heard a sympathetic apology. I felt remorse, but my survival instinct prevailed. I kept moving.

Several weeks later we heard from Barbara's daughter. She and her husband had returned to Washington State to live happily ever after while Barbara and I had made our way to Palm Springs, California.

Barbara's daughter relayed a story that a friend of her husband had told concerning a blind man with a cane causing him to fall on his face in the casino.

Now I ask you, what are the odds? If I had known those odds were with me on that occasion, I would have taken my chances at the roulette wheel.

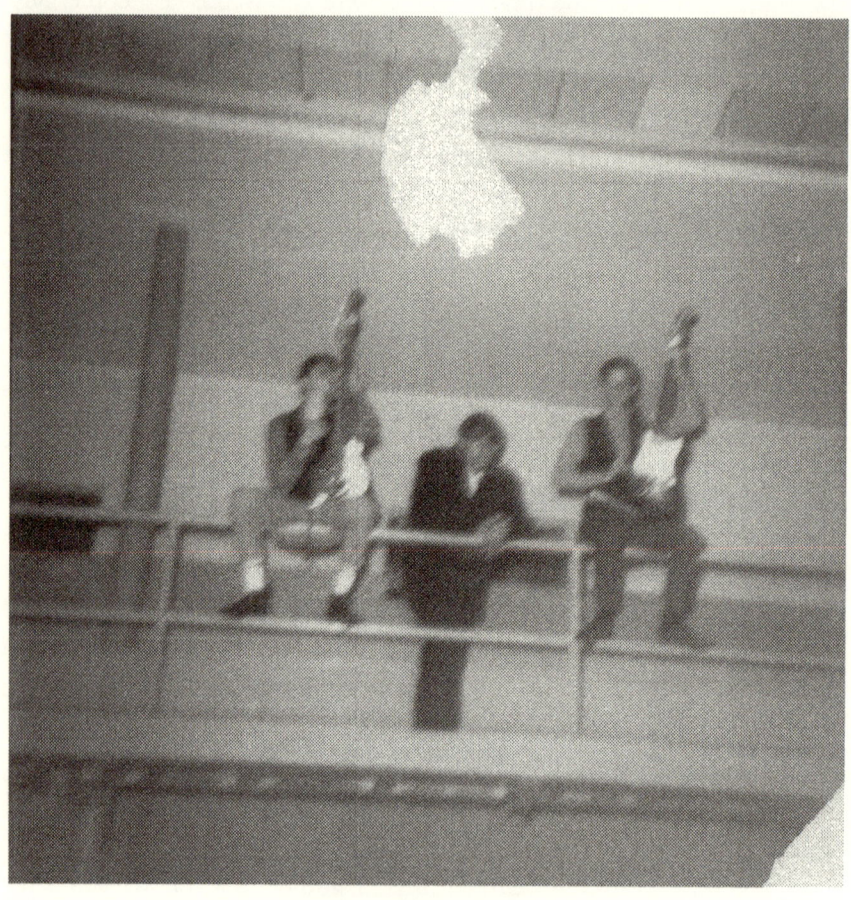

My first band, "The Vibrations" -
Eminence, Missouri 1966 - High School Gym
Left to right, Michael, John Counts and Robert Deel

Chapter 7
California Dreamin'

In 1969 I took my first hit of LSD. Some guy on campus asked me if I wanted to drop some acid. I said, "Sure, why not?" Not only did I not know that acid was LSD but I had no idea that my life would be changed forever. The guy placed a tablet in my hand about the size of a match head. I remember thinking to myself, "What can this do to me? It's so small." Well, I was soon to find out.

My fellow travelers and I lay prostrate on the floor for hours. We had no concept of time. We were not only listening to the music pouring from the stereo, we could also see it. The music was every color of the rainbow. It was a beautiful experience, and I still believe it to be a turning point in my life. Words fail to describe it. It's comparable to explaining an orgasm to a virgin. Please don't misunderstand. I am not advocating the use of drugs, but I firmly believe that the LSD trip was a catalyst for events to come.

A few weeks after my psychedelic journey, I removed myself from academia and promptly declared my freedom by hitch-hiking to California. My curiosity about the hippie culture on the West Coast had finally gotten the best of me, and it was time to act.

Sometimes sleep escapes me when I think of the California endeavor, for like most young people, I knew not the meaning of fear. I could see no better at night at the age of nineteen than I can now thirty-five years later. I could only see lights. My depth perception has always been excellent, so I could accurately judge the distance between myself and a moving vehicle. Also, I could tell when I was on the pavement or the shoulder of the road by the feelings and sounds beneath my feet.

I traveled to Oakland, California, before I encountered a potential disaster. I was given a ride by a man driving a Mustang fastback. In those days this was known as a "muscle car." I was somewhat experienced with hot rods, so when he became fatigued from driving and asked me if I wanted to take the wheel, I was thrilled.

It was fun. The combination of rock'n'roll on the radio and the roar and feel of the big engine was exciting to a wild and crazy young man such as myself. It was my first time to experience the Wild West. I cruised for a couple of hundred miles at speeds approaching 100 miles an hour.

However, as we neared Oakland the mood and the terrain began to radically change.

I was about to be introduced to a thing called a FREEWAY. I can assure you that had I known what it was like to drive on a freeway, I would never have allowed myself to be caught in that crazy, nerve-wracking situation.

Let me describe the situation for you. I was in ten lanes of traffic. There were five going to Oakland and five coming from God knows where and no vehicle was doing less than 80 miles an hour. Hell, it was like one massive race, thousands of cars rolling around curves and over hills. To make matters worse, there was no guard rail or concrete divide to help prevent five lanes of traffic, each going in the opposite direction, from smashing into each other.

Yours truly was driving in the lane nearest the on-coming traffic, and guess what, Mom and Dad? IT WAS GETTING DARK. I casually asked the dude who owned the car if he was ready to drive. I didn't have the heart to tell the poor bastard that a guy was driving his car at break-neck speed in the middle of a freeway and would soon be "visually impaired," as the politically correct idiots are so fond of saying.

It was time to get off the freeway, but not only had I not driven on a freeway, I had not had the experience of exiting one. Californians would soon give me a lesson I would not soon forget.

I immediately switched my right turn signal on to alert other drivers that it was my intention to change lanes. I assumed that was the proper thing to do. I am sure that many of them just smiled and shook their head in disbelief, saying to themselves "That poor guy. Does he really think we're gonna slow down and let him into our lane? He must be a hillbilly from the Ozarks." They refused to allow me to change lanes, and by now I was rapidly losing precious daylight.

I was growing concerned, but when people began to switch on their headlights this nineteen-year-old blind hippie hillbilly began to panic.

I was becoming desperate. With my right arm I began waving people back. Once again they totally ignored my signals. By now I was not only scared; I was becoming agitated to the point of profanity.

You should have seen the look on the guy's face who owned the car I was driving. His eyes were so wide he looked like Bart Simpson or Little Orphan Annie. I said, "Man, I'm not kidding, we've got to find an exit and get the hell off this freeway because I have night blindness and if we don't we're in big trouble!"

Remember my buddy David Beck that was on the back of the motorcycle? Well, this guy's reaction was quite similar. He sat motionless with a blank look on his face and uttered not one word.

I was desperate. I had no intention of ending my life because of these rude idiots on the freeway. I began to use the automobile I was piloting to get their attention. It weighed several thousand pounds and was traveling at a high rate of speed, so if that didn't work, nothing would.

At just the right moment I would weave across the dividing line and then return to my lane. At first even this maneuver failed to get their attention, but eventually those crazy Californians realized that the cat in the Mustang might just be something to back away from.

This technique proved successful, but it took about twenty minutes to exit the freeway. When I stepped from the car I was once again shaking like a whore in church. My driving skills from being a hot rodder in the Ozark Mountains had certainly paid off, and with not a minute to spare, for by the time we exited the freeway it was dusk, and headlights and street lamps were all I could see.

I thought I had learned my lesson. From this point on I would make certain that if I drove, I would relinquish the wheel at least one hour before the sun would sink beneath that great western sky. In other words, I would cover my ass.

Once again I was in unfamiliar territory, and man, you just don't know what's around the next corner. A day or two after the freeway incident I was driving another car and feeling quite confident, having successfully avoided a potential disaster. I was running along about 80 miles an hour, just cruising and listening to the radio with not a care in the world. If someone would try to plan a bad dream for a person with night blindness they could never improve upon what loomed in front of me. It was a TUNNEL.

It took a few seconds to register. I couldn't believe it. I had no options. What was I to do? I was in the middle of traffic and there was no escape.

As we entered the tunnel I remember thinking, "This is it! I'm going to die right here!" We went from bright sunlight to pitch black in one second. It was exactly like the caves I explored as a child but with one huge difference. I was driving a vehicle at 80 miles an hour in the middle of a goddamned California freeway, and I was about to be totally blind.

We entered the tunnel and total darkness. Never before had I felt such complete terror. I tried to keep my cool as I held the wheel steady, expecting to hear and feel a crash at any moment. Just as I felt I could not stifle a scream, there it was. It was so beautiful. It was a light at the end of the tunnel. It was rapidly getting larger. I could see the silhouette of cars ahead of me. Before I knew it we were in the glorious sunlight. Thank you so much, Blind Fairy.

The poor bastard sitting next to me had no idea just how close he came to shaking hands with the Grim Reaper. From that point on, I let someone else do the driving.

After three days I reached Berkeley, California, from Springfield, Missouri. I arrived at my destination without a hitch, if you will pardon the pun.

After roaming the west for a few weeks and having satisfied my curiosity, I decided it was time to go home.

The return trip was going fine until I reached Oklahoma. It was around three a.m., and I was standing on what I thought was the shoulder of the road when I noticed a tractor trailer truck coming toward me, frantically honking his horn. I thought he was just giving me shit, because believe me, in those days hippies got their share. It was within a few hundred yards from me when I noticed that something was very wrong. I was directly in its path.

At the last moment I leaped to safety. I was three feet from oblivion. The force of the speeding truck left me on my hippie hillbilly ass at the edge of the road. Luckily my suitcase also escaped injury. Thanks again, Blind Fairy.

There is a perpetual wind in Oklahoma, so that would probably account for the gravel on the pavement. It could also be said that exhaustion had a hand in this, but I can tell you, from that moment on Michael was very attentive.

An hour or so later and a few miles closer to home it was not yet daylight, and I was wearily standing by the road praying for a ride, when from behind me I heard what sounded like someone or some thing making its way through the brush.

I heard a deep, masculine, confident voice speaking to me. Immediately I could tell it was a black man. I would not be lying if I told you I damned near passed out from fright. He said, "What's happenin', man?"

We walked along for a couple of hours trying to hitch a ride. There was much conversation. He had been traveling the highways and railroads of America for sixty years. I asked a thousand questions.

That old man had nothing more than what he could carry, but he had something very valuable. It's called "inner peace," and I will never forget him. During this encounter I learned lessons not taught in a classroom, and I will be forever grateful to him for not chopping this blind hippie hillbilly's ass up into little pieces.

I am aware of the danger I exposed myself to by hitch-hiking to California at the tender age of nineteen and not being able to see a damned thing at night, but I would not trade that experience for anything. It was a crash course in life, although you couldn't pay me enough money to do it today. It's a different world. I left Springfield with eight dollars in my pocket and returned with four. In those days all you had to have was some hair and maybe a pair of wire-rimmed glasses and you were part of the revolution. People took care of each other. The movement didn't last long, but I am very grateful to have played my part in it. My job was to play my guitar and make love with the rock'n'roll mamas. It was a tough job, but someone had to do it.

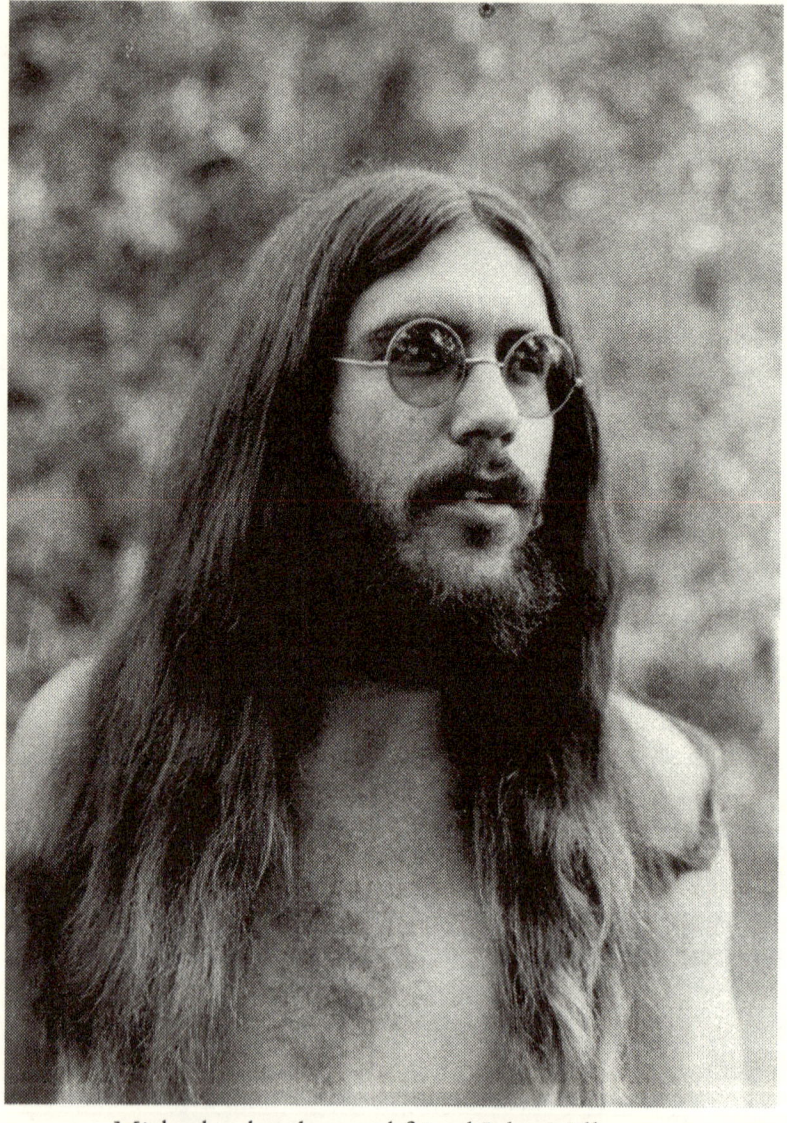

Michael, taken by good friend John Miller

Chapter 8
Blind Man Running

I'll never forget my first jog. In 1969 my good friend Michael Libertus had a wife. This wife happened to be majoring in physical education at SMS in Springfield, Missouri.

After much coaxing they finally managed to drag me to the track. Years earlier I had been quite proficient at running. Street gangs had, if you recall, been the primary source of motivation. I jogged twice around the quarter mile track, if you could call it jogging, and I thought I would die. My lungs were on fire and I was weak and trembling.

Well, this would never do. For God's sake, I was nineteen years of age. Call it ego or self preservation, I don't know, but come hell or high water I would never again allow myself to deteriorate to such a degree.

Through the years I reached a higher level of discipline. Jogging became an integral part of my life. In the beginning my vision was not an issue, but as the years rolled by and it worsened, it gradually became something I had to deal with. Jogging was something I loved, especially in the country.

Naturally jogging in the country on gravel roads was much easier. Sure, I would split mud puddles from time to time, but that was no big deal. I've often considered myself fortunate that I didn't step on a poisonous snake, or any kind of snake for that matter, since this would almost certainly have induced heart failure.

I jogged my way through the '70s and most of the '80s before things began to happen. I had tunnel vision, and as the opening of the tunnel diminished I had to pay close attention to my surroundings, especially in the city.

One day around 1988 I was jogging from my house to Phelps Grove Park in Springfield, a route I had jogged many times. There was a small curb dividing the street from the park. The curb had never been a problem, but this time was different. As my foot found the obstacle I knew instantly I was in trouble with no chance of recovery. I made a split-second decision to do a somersault. As I fell forward I tucked in, and the next thing that hit the ground was the back of my head. The momentum carried me forward, and I rolled to my feet without missing a step.

Not only was I unharmed, but my self esteem was intact. That particular patch of ground was free of roots and rock, or the outcome may have been totally different. A sane person with such visual impairment would have purchased a tread mill that day, but as you may have guessed by now, I just don't do things the easy way.

A few years later, just a 100 yards from the location of the miraculous somersault, I was jogging on a beautiful, crisp October day and feeling great. I bounded over the infamous curve without missing a step. There was a path around the park worn from years of jogging, walking, and other activities, and this was easy to follow.

They had dug a ditch around the park to bury an electric line. This ran parallel to the path. I had to jump the ditch to get to the path as I had done for several days with no problem. I jumped the ditch and the momentum carried me several steps beyond the path. As I leaped the ditch I was also leaping from sunlight to shade. That's when it happened. There was a bright, flashing light, then total darkness. My mind could not comprehend what had happened.

There were voices, concerned and anxious. "Are you okay?" They were repeating this question to me, but I was unable to answer.

As I slowly regained my senses it became apparent that, as had happened many times in my life, my eyesight had once again failed me. I became aware of my surroundings as they were helping me to my feet. They found my glasses and were genuinely concerned.

As you must know by now I am an old pro at facing embarrassing situations in which I would find myself because of my poor vision. I brushed myself off and thanked the good citizens for their help. I would not, however, endeavor to explain why I had slammed face-first into a tree while jogging. This would take much too long, and after all, I would most likely never see these people again.

I have to laugh out loud when I think of all the poor bastards I have confounded with my antics over the years. Now can you imagine taking a stroll in the park on a beautiful day and witnessing some guy run face first into a tree? I would love to know what goes through their minds when they see something like that. I would laugh my ass off. I was so happy the only injury I sustained was a knot between my eyes that I promise you I really didn't give a shit what anyone thought.

Those who know me well can tell you that I would not choose a dog as my best friend, so dog lovers out there should enjoy the humor and irony to be found on the following pages. As I have stated I loved to jog in the country. I had been jogging past the farm of Fuzz Smith for at least twenty-five years. The farm is located on the Jack's Fork River just below Eminence, Missouri.

On this particular day a big black dog belonging to Bebe Bryant, the mother of my twin daughters, decided to accompany me. At first I liked the idea. It was nice to jog and have a companion. For years I had seen yuppies jog with their loyal pets running beside them. I would say to myself, "Man, these people are such idiots," but I must say, it felt pretty good.

I was jogging at a pretty good clip past Fuzz Smith's house. He was working in his yard, and I waved as I always had, and that's when it happened.

The dog had decided to cut in front of me. With no peripheral vision, the inevitable happened.

I suppose you could call it "doggie justice," for Michael McIntire went sprawling down the middle of the gravel road. I rolled and tumbled, skinning myself up pretty good. I'll bet Fuzz and that dog were grinning from ear to ear.

As usual, I tried to hide my embarrassment. I promptly got up and looked around as I brushed myself off. Since I felt like a fool, it's reasonable to assume that I would say something foolish. I said, "I'm gonna kill that damned dog."

Standing there with a smile on his face and thoroughly enjoying himself, Fuzz said, "Looks like he's gonna kill you first."

At that moment hillbilly humor was the last thing I wanted to hear, but through the years as I have reconstructed the incident in my mind, I have laughed out loud. On a recent walk which took us past the Fuzz Smith Farm, my lady, Sandie Zemblidge, and I had the good fortune to visit with the eighty-three-year-old farmer. It had been twenty-five years since the dog had tried to kill me, and as I asked him about it I was curious. Would he remember?

"Oh yeah" he said, "seems to me that dog got the better of you that day." I could not see him, but I am certain he was still wearing that same grin and I'm sure his dogs were also smiling.

For the last thirty years my parents have owned a cabin on the Current River. A five mile stretch of gravel road off Highway 19 north of Eminence takes you there. I am certain I have jogged hundreds of miles on that road over the years. In the beginning it was easy, but these days the light is brighter where the road is, and that's the only way I can tell where I am.

It was about a year ago (2003) during the winter. I was spending a few days at the cabin alone, just getting away from it all.

I went for my daily jog and I had gotten a late start. It was around three o'clock in the afternoon. It would get dark at five, so I assumed I would have more than enough time.

I was returning to the cabin when I sensed something wrong. The road didn't feel the same under my feet. Also, the angle of the light was different. I kept jogging, but I was growing concerned.

Then I saw an orange blur directly ahead. I slowed to a walk and cautiously approached the orange object. It was a gate and the orange thing was a government sign. This meant that several miles back I had taken a wrong turn.

My first impulse was to panic. I was alone in the woods by myself, couldn't see shit, the temperature was already below freezing, and darkness was approaching. Of course I would backtrack, but if I took another wrong turn I could easily be stranded, exposed to the elements. My greatest concern was the falling temperature.

It's during a situation such as this that I hear the voices of my loved ones. They say things like, "You have no business out there alone trying to jog, anything could happen to you," and I begin to doubt myself.

I begin to think, "Wow! Maybe they are right, maybe I am crazy for being in the woods alone." When I have this discussion with myself it is always a short one, and invariably I will come to the same conclusion. I did not ask to be born, but having been dropped on this planet, as long as I live I will enjoy life. I love the outdoors, and I refuse to live my life in fear.

As I tried to make my way back to the cabin in the middle of winter, miles from the nearest human being, fear hung over me like a wet blanket. I was scared shitless.

Retracing my steps, I had been jogging for about 30 minutes when I began to notice that the amount of light had increased and the road was in better condition. To my right the sun was setting behind the Ozark Mountains. (The sun was the only thing I could see).

My mind was racing. I was trying to stay calm, and then it hit me. When traveling to the cabin the sun is always on my left. I would notice something like this because the sun is all I can see.

I immediately reversed direction, but if you'll pardon the pun I was not out of the woods yet. It was almost dark, and I had at least three miles to go.

In case you are wondering, it's easy to stay on the road, because the gravel changes. In other words, it's thicker at the edge and in the middle, because of traffic. It's a subtle feeling beneath your feet, but if you pay close attention, this method will work. However, I have yet to figure out a warning system for fallen branches, etc.

When I began to jog down a long, steep hill I knew that I was close to the river. I was cold and pissed off.

I do not want to give the impression that I run fast. Hell, I'm blind, not stupid. I just lope along like an old wolf, but I was making time. There was one more fork in the road, but if I made the right turn I would be home free.

Well guess what, once again, I took the road leading nowhere. By now it was almost totally dark, and man, was it cold.

I backtracked again and used some good old-fashioned deductive reasoning. I knew that if I started jogging uphill again I would be taking myself further from the river. "DUH!" I had to turn right, so I kept to the right, and as I jogged I was feeling better about things, except for the fact that I was freezing my hippie hillbilly ass off.

Finally, I heard a most welcome sound, the sound of water, and at that moment I have never heard "Current River" sound better. I knew that our cabin is located at the only point along the river where you can hear the water making its wonderful music.

Being almost completely blind I do not fear darkness, and it's a damned good thing, for by now I was surrounded by it.

Over the years Craft Road, which leads to our cabin, has gone through some changes. When I first began jogging on that road it was pretty rough. It was narrow, there were many pot holes, and the traffic was slight—sometimes only one or two cars a day.

Well, that's not the case today, baby. When I jog on that road today, just for old times' sake, I will encounter at least two or three vehicles. (Last deer season I counted seventeen during my jog.) The government has widened the road extensively, and these days it is well maintained. So this means that like the rest of the country, everyone is driving three times faster than is necessary. I can hear them coming long before they get to me. When they approach I hit the ditch. Sometimes they are running 40 or 50 miles an hour, which is why these days I do most of my jogging on the tread mill.

The "Little Old Lady Incident" took place in Phelps Grove Park in 1995, shortly before the devastating wreck in which I was nearly killed. (I will write more of this in the following pages.)

I knew that my days of jogging in the city were numbered. There was just too much going on for me to keep track of with my tunnel vision. It was like looking through a tube, and the tube was getting smaller. Because of my apprehension it was no longer enjoyable. However, I was hanging in there, and like most people, I would resist change.

I was jogging on the path that surrounds the park, and as usual, I steadily scanned the area with my limited vision, trying to avoid running into something, most notably trees.

I saw two people at the other end of the park. There was no problem, for I was keeping a sharp eye on them. Yeah right, the legally blind guy was keeping a sharp eye on them, all right. (I used to be an outlaw. I was illegally blind but they busted me, and now I'm a card carrying blind citizen.)

I jogged along thinking I had everything covered. As I grew closer to the people, I could see they were not on the path. I could also see they were a couple of little old ladies, and they were just standing there talking. I kept jogging.

Suddenly my feet became tangled in something. This fried my brain for I had no clue of what was happening. Each time I tried to place my foot in front of me I was stepping on something soft and pliable. At first I thought, "Jesus Christ! Not another damned dog." As I fell forward I smacked into something heavy and warm. Instinctively I reached out, and as I did so my hands grasped someone's shoulders.

I heard a small, weak voice exclaim, "Oh my God!"

Instantly my brain grasped the situation. I thought, "Well, you're in deep shit now, McIntire. Not only are you riding piggy-back on a little old lady, but if you live through this, it's gonna be litigation city."

The piggy-back ride only lasted for a few seconds, but I swear it seemed to go on forever. I was stumbling forward and trying to keep her from falling at the same time. Each time I tried to take a step some part of the poor woman's body was under my feet. Hell, if she didn't have a heart attack, why not finish her off by trampling her to death?

It was hopeless. I couldn't save us. She was not a frail, petite granny. She weighed at least 200 pounds.

Now we were on the ground, and I was on top of her. Doesn't that paint a picture? Hell, the more I tried to get off her, the more I wallowed her. I just knew I was killing her.

I finally made it to my feet and helped her stand. I felt so sorry for this woman I wanted to cry. There she was, walking along, minding her own business, and some blind hippie hillbilly runs her into the ground.

I wanted to crawl into a hole and pull the dirt in after me. I was ready to take my cussin', and then call an ambulance for her.

I couldn't believe what happened next.

SHE ASKED ME IF I WAS OKAY. I was in shock. I've never apologized to someone so many times and with such sincerity in my life. She kept saying, "It's all right honey."

I was so relieved she wasn't hurt, it was hard to concentrate. She was talking to me, but I wasn't hearing her. I told her of my vision problems, and she then proceeded to tell me of her son-in-law's poor eyesight.

We stood there in the park and conversed for about 20 minutes. Man, at that moment, if that woman would have asked me if I would cut my hair and become a preacher, I would have told her to point me to the pulpit.

For a few months after the "Little Old Lady Incident" I continued to jog around the park, although I must say, I did this with great caution. Then the wreck happened, and the decision to stop jogging in the park was no longer mine.

For months following the wreck I would walk around the park. My recovery was slow, and I was never alone. I would never jog in the city again, and truthfully I don't miss it, for if a blind man is going to jog he should consider doing so in the country, where it's unlikely he will encounter a little old lady, but damned likely he will encounter a copperhead. Stay tuned.

From 1995 through 2002 I jogged on a tread mill. Then I returned once again to my roots. I was back in "Booger County" and my beloved Ozark Mountains.

God! How I looked forward to trotting over those beautiful hills.

Knowing their son, my parents promptly admonished, "You're not jogging the roads alone." As usual I did not argue, but merely smiled, for nothing on God's green earth would stop me. At no time have I felt more alive than when out there on a warm spring day, making love with Mother Nature.

A couple of times a week my mother, Nina McIntire, would take me to Craft Road, the road leading to the cabin. I would get out at the beginning of the gravel road, and she would wait for me about 2 ½ miles ahead. We followed this routine for about a year with no major problems.

Sometimes after a storm there would be the inevitable tree limb that had blown across the road. I would be jogging along, and suddenly I would feel the tips of the branches, and having been there, done that, I would immediately come to a halt, but not before finding myself wading through the middle of a tree. There were times when the tree was large, but it was usually rotten. Having had experience with such things I can testify that if you're going to run into a tree, run into a rotten one.

This tale is so poignant I must share it with you. It was one of those bright, crisp, sunny days. It was very quiet, for there was no breeze, and I was jogging on the Craft Road. My breathing and footsteps on the gravel were all my sensitive hearing could detect until I heard something at a great distance. I am accustomed to hearing animals scamper through the woods as I jog along, but this was different. It was big.

At first I could hardly hear it, but with each second the sound grew louder. I slowed to a walk, listening intently. I could tell that it was moving fast as it literally bounced through the woods. Immediately I knew it was a deer, and I thought, "Man! This thing's gonna run over me."

I stopped and listened as it approached. It must have seen me or caught my scent, (poor deer) for it bounded across the road about 30 feet ahead of me.

I knew it had crossed the road, because with each stride I could hear its hooves as they made contact with the leaves. When it jumped the road there was dead silence. It was awesome. The only sound was that of its hooves hitting the middle of the road.

I do not wish for eyesight often, but on this occasion I would have loved to have had the ability to see, if only for a few seconds. If this sounds trivial to you, imagine being blindfolded in the wilderness and something large is running in your direction.

In 2003 I finally realized a dream of thirty years. I bought a house in the Ozark Mountains with one road leading in. This road is roughly one-half mile long. The road I am speaking of runs from the highway to my house.

Again I found myself without access to a tread-mill, but as I had been jogging for thirty-four years and a jogging addict, I just had to give it a try.

Unlike the Craft Road, the road which leads to my house is extremely narrow and rough. I used my official white cane issued to me by the government (after all, I am now "legally blind") and walked to the highway and back a few times just to check things out.

Finally I gave it a try. It was difficult from the beginning. One step off the road and you were in the brush. It was nerve wracking.

Sometimes after a rain the road became slick. At the edge of the road where the grader had been it was scooped out like a bowl. More than once I found myself flat on my ass, and I hadn't fallen in years.

Once while jogging, and after having progressed several hundred yards from my house when, veering from the road, I scratched my leg on some barbed wire. This would not do. I had to change my method of operation or abstain from my jog. The latter was not an option.

For years people would teasingly ask me if I jogged with a white cane. With my usual smartass come back I would retort, "Hell yes," but now I was ready to try anything.

I grabbed my trusty cane and we set off. I hadn't gone far when I knew I was on to something. As I jogged I would sweep the cane from left to right, and back again. I was cutting a swath about eight feet on either side and ahead of me.

If I strayed left or right the cane would come in contact with vegetation. Hell, if I would attach a blade to the cane, I could cut brush and jog simultaneously. Some of my smartass friends had the nerve to tell me that my driveway had grown wider. Don't worry, I knew it was untrue. Remember, I'm blind, not stupid, although that case could be argued.

With this new procedure I cut three minutes off my jogging time, plus it was far less hazardous. However, I did jog onto Highway 19 several times, but I can assure you this error was corrected immediately.

During the summer of 2003 my housekeeper, Melba Shipton, ran over a 3 1/2 foot timber rattler while driving from my house to the highway. The tread mill was sounding better every day.

As of January 2004 I am the proud owner of a tread mill. Occasionally, I will jog on the Craft Road for sentimental reasons, for I hope to continue to be a "Blind Man Running."

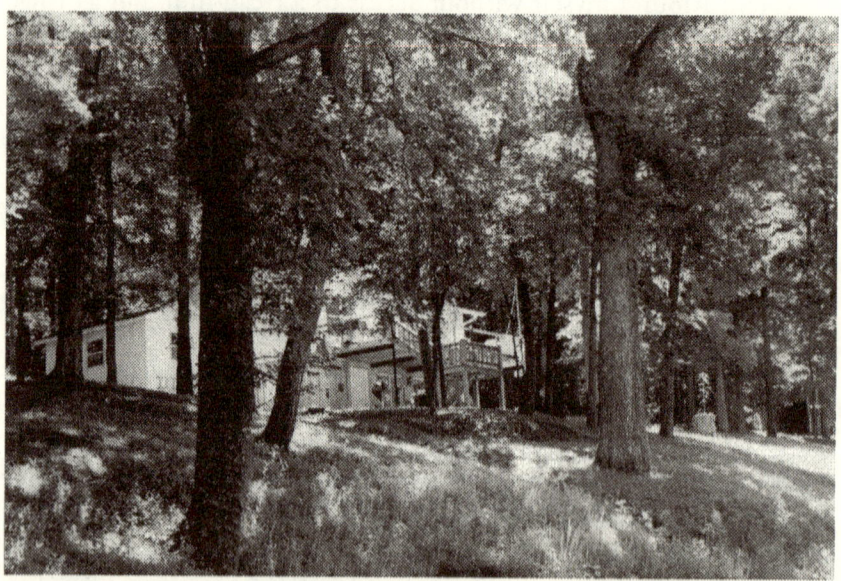

The Cabin on Current River

Chapter 9
On the Road Again

In June of 1999 Barbara Hoskin and I set out on the road playing music. After having a near-death experience in 1995 (the wreck), I made the decision to shake things up. It was one of the most exciting undertakings of my life. We had no idea what lay before us, but the two of us were adventurous people, and we would give it our best shot.

We spent the summer of 1998 in the Lake Tahoe, Nevada area, where most of the time I managed to avoid trouble, but as luck would have it, I would find myself in situations such as the "Retarded Guy Incident."

Barbara and I had just played a gig at a biker bar in the middle of the afternoon in Virginia City and we were starving, so we headed across the street to the Red Dog Saloon to get a bite to eat.

We strolled to the counter to place our order. We had been there many times and knew the employees. I was standing there, spaced out as usual, while Barbara spoke with the guy behind the counter. As I began to slowly tune in to the conversation I couldn't believe what I was hearing. She was helping this guy spell words a third-grader could handle, and then to my amazement, they began to add numbers.

We're not talking large sums, they were single digit numbers.

Man, I thought I was dreaming, and then I realized the guy behind the counter was speaking as a retarded guy would.

I thought, "This is ridiculous, if they think I'm gonna fall for this bullshit, they're crazy." What person in their right mind would hire a guy whose guitar is not in tune to work in an eating establishment?

Now I'm not going to lie to you. I had been drinking a little whiskey, and I am sure that only added to the confusion. I always warn people, "The only thing worse than a blind man on the loose is a drunk blind man on the loose."

I had befriended some crazy people in Virginia City since my arrival, and like the rest of my crazy friends around the country, they liked to mess with the blind guy. Well, I was not going to fall for it.

I've always done a pretty good imitation of a retarded guy, and I had sipped enough whiskey to be uncertain as to whether or not I was faking it, but I fell into character. I would play along. As I gave my order I was slurring my words and franticly waving my arms in the air as I thought a retarded guy might do.

As we two retarded guys tried to communicate Barbara was elbowing me in the ribs and dragging me away from the scene. I failed to understand her reaction, for after all, I have a sense of humor. I was just playing along with the joke.

When we had seated ourselves at a table she proceeded to explain the situation to me, and as she did so, I slumped in my chair. The guy wasn't faking it.

He was definitely mentally challenged, and as it turns out, the son of the proprietor.

His parents were old, spaced out hippies. Hell, they were older than me, and I'm so old the Dead Sea was just sick when I was born.

I don't know what these people were thinking, but in order to put their retarded son in the position of running the cash register, they must have been taking some damned good drugs.

First I run a little old lady down, and then I make fun of a retarded guy. What next?

I couldn't win because, if I apologized, I'm reasonably certain that he would not have understood what the hell I was saying, and I would certainly not try to explain this to his parents.

I am the last person in the world to make fun of an impaired person, so I took the only option left to me. I ate my pizza and then got the hell out of Dodge.

About a week later, I would engage in a one- way conversation with someone possessing my level of intelligence.

Barbara and I were on the outskirts of Virginia City, and in need of directions, we rolled along side an officer of the law, seated in his patrol car. As I lowered my window, and began my inquiry, Barbara attempted to interrupt. Impatiently, I said, "Wait just a minute dear," and continued conversing with the constable.

Appropriately, Barbara shrugged, and let Mr. Mac dig himself a big hole. After a time, I began to notice something was not quite right. I was doing all of the talking. When I would pause, there was an uncomfortable silence. Finally, I turned to Barbara and asked, "What the hell is going on? Is he taking a snooze?"

She had attempted to inform me of the situation, but I had refused to heed the warning.

It seems the good People of Virginia City, had planted a decoy, with a dummy, attired in patrolman's hat, official uniform, etc., in hopes of reminding people of their speedometer.

The joke may have been on me, but I got a hell of a good laugh out of it, and I think it's an ingenious idea. However, if they would have tried that trick in Shannon county, during the 60's, it would have been necessary to get officer Dummy home by sundown, or by sun up, he would have had so many holes in him, he would have had to seek employment as a scarecrow.

I can tell you from experience, when you get impaired people together, anything can happen. When I have occasion to be introduced to another blind person, sometimes it takes us fifteen minutes to shake hands, which brings me to my next story.

In the early 90s Debbie Hediger and I were playing music in Houston, Missouri, when once again this blind boy put on quite a show for the folks, and I'm not just referring to singing and playing the guitar.

We were relaxing while on break and conversing with a few of the locals when I remarked that I would like to dance, but I found myself without a partner.

I was in luck, for sitting across the table from me was a guy who could match me at being a smartass any day of the week. He said, "I'll dance with ya." Having had a few drinks, I said, "Let's go."

Hell, I'll do anything for a laugh, but so you don't get the wrong impression, it was not a slow dance; I mean, we weren't in love or anything. We were a hit. I could hear people laughing and applauding.

As we returned to our seat I endeavored to shake hands with him and offer my congratulations on what a fine dance it was, but there was no response. I stood there for a moment with my hand in front of me. Realizing my efforts were futile, I slowly took my place in the booth.

Once again I was the last to know. At the appropriate time Debbie informed me the guy had no arms.

Oh, what a beautiful picture comes to mind. It's no wonder people were laughing and applauding. Not only were two guys dancing, but one was blind, and the other had no arms. For an encore we stood facing each other while I tried to shake hands with the poor bastard.

He was quite a guy and was blessed with a hell of a sense of humor. He later told the story of losing his arms.

He was electrocuted while at the top of a pole trying to steal copper from a transformer. While I usually have no sympathy for thieves, his punishment was a bit harsh. I hope to meet him again some day, and if I do, I will ask him if he would like to take our little act on the road.

A few months before the wreck in 1995 Debbie and I were doing a gig at the Golden Lounge, where we had been the house band for about a year. We were familiar with most of the regulars. It was a slow night, and I was sitting in a booth on break.

Suddenly I was approached, and someone began waving their hands in front of my face and making weird sounds. There were hisses and whistles along with moans and grunts. It reminded me of a horror movie.

I thought, "Here we go again, one of my dear friends messin' with the blind man." So I did what I always do. I played along.

He was poking me in the chest, making those god-awful sounds and slobbering on me, so I started doing the same thing to him.

We were quite the entertainers. People were losing it, and the more they laughed, the more I played along.

Much to my relief he grew weary of this game and moved along, whereupon Debbie plopped down beside me, and finally catching her breath from laughter, proceeded to paint the picture.

He was truly a friend, and it was no trick. He was a deaf guy simply trying to convey to me how much he enjoyed my music. I wanted to crawl under the table.

He had been a fan of mine for years, but he hadn't been around for a while.

It was like the movie with Gene Wilder and Richard Pryor, "Hear No Evil, See No Evil." A deaf guy and a blind guy can get into lots of trouble in a short time.

While living in the Lake Tahoe area, we resided in an RV park in Carson City. One morning during my usual routine of sunning and drinking coffee, a little old lady next door said, "It's a beautiful day isn't it?" Summoning all of my southern charm, I returned her pleasant, unsolicited greeting by saying, "Yes ma'am, it certainly is." I could hear her puttering in her yard, and after a moment of silence I said, "Have you lived here long?" There was no reply. Thinking my question unheard, I repeated it. Again there was no reply. I simply shrugged and returned to my contemplation of sun and coffee.

Later that evening as I expressed my bewilderment at the strange behavior of our neighbor, Barbara said, "Well, Mac, you've done it again."

She proceeded to explain to me that our neighbor was far from being a little old lady. In fact she was a man, and this man was in his late thirties.

I should take this opportunity to point out that I am not now, nor have I ever been, prejudiced against gay people. As long as they leave me alone I don't care what the hell they do, and I feel that way toward everyone. In other words; "live and let live!"

It seems the gay guy was an employee of the RV Park. He cleaned restrooms. I would later discover that he was heavy into drugs and was a chain smoker. This would account for the deep, raspy voice. They told me he looked like death warmed over.

Being from the Midwest I hadn't been around many gay people, but I would soon further my education.

The fact that I had mistaken a young, homosexual male for a little old lady would not in itself be of much interest, but this would not be the conclusion of the story.

Two years would pass before our road trip would, once more, take Barbara and me to the Lake Tahoe area. Having friends in Carson City, we chose to live in the same RV park as before.

On a sunny, windy western day I was again sitting on the patio when I heard footsteps, as a person was walking on the street in front of me. A voice said, "It's a beautiful day isn't it?"

"Yes, ma'am, it certainly is," I replied. I made another attempt at conversation, but the person walked on in silence.

Several minutes passed as I thought of nothing in particular; then I happened to recall that the footsteps led to the public restrooms, about 300 yards from me.

It was then that my deductive reasoning kicked in. It hit me like a ton of bricks. I thought, "No! This can't be happening to me twice in one lifetime, and involving the same person."

That evening I learned that it truly was my (little old lady-gay guy) friend, and he, she, it, whatever, had maintained employment as a restroom specialist for the RV park.

If he was as drugged out as they said, it was unlikely that he would recollect our previous encounter of two years hence. As I have stated, a person's sexual preference is of no interest to me, but in my view, if laws can be passed pertaining to everything from spitting on the sidewalk to forcing an adult to protect his or her own skull by wearing a helmet while riding a motorcycle, then, by God, a law should be passed forcing gay people to identify themselves to blind people.

This could be accomplished with the use of special audio devices such as beepers, bells, etc. No cards or letters please.

It was also during our second pass through the Lake Tahoe area that, while playing music at a place called Fly's Silver Dollar Saloon in Virginia City, I would have my second encounter with a person of mixed gender in the Wild, Wild West. We had played a couple of sets and were taking a break. I was sitting at the bar with an elderly couple and the bartender making casual conversation. As I returned to the stage the elderly gentleman paid for a drink and had it delivered to me.

As I began my next set I remembered the appropriate manners Mother had taught me and spoke into the microphone thanking the patron and his spouse for the tasty beverage. I could sense the levity in the room, but the humor of the comment escaped me.

About 30 minutes later as I was finishing a song, everyone in the bar surrounded the stage. They were laughing their asses off. I had done it again.

The bartender told me that when I had thanked them for the drink using the microphone (meaning that everyone in the room would hear the comment), the guy that I assumed was the husband turned to the bartender and said, "He really can't see, can he?" This would explain the mild laughter I had heard.

It was a couple of gay men, and this blind hippie hillbilly was the only person in the damned room that didn't have a clue. Case in point: if they would have been wearing the worldwide standardized gay bell, I would have known what was going on along with everyone else in the room.

This would explain why everyone had waited until the cowboy sweethearts had departed to let "yours truly" in on the joke.

The incident is still talked about in Virginia City, but I still can't get over the fact that I could mistake a gay guy for a little old lady. That scares the hell out of me. Until they make gay bells mandatory, it would probably be much safer for this blind boy to just continue to wander the Ozark Mountains.

In October of 1999, as the weather grew colder in the Lake Tahoe area, we, being snow-songbirds, packed up and headed for Palm Springs, California. We soon procured a gig at T's Roadhouse in Cathedral City, California, a small town bordering Palm Springs. In the Palm Springs area there are about six towns bordering each other. You can't tell where one ends and the other begins. Why they don't consolidate is beyond my understanding.

After playing a few eating establishments, country clubs, etc., quite naturally we landed a gig at a place known to raise hell. T's Roadhouse was a biker bar. Wow! I was just like Jeff Healey, the blind musician in the movie *Roadhouse*.

During that winter we made good music and many friends. The place rocked. Not surprisingly, motorcycles were the main topic of conversation, and sometimes after knocking back a few I would fondly return to the "good old days" when I myself straddled the "iron steed."

One night I was telling tales of my riding adventures to an old veteran biker, Ponytail Terry, and I'm not talking about a weekend warrior. This cat was the real thing. He was around long before doctors and lawyers decided to get on the Harley band wagon and perch their pretty little wives and girlfriends on the leather seat in their cute little short shorts.

I was crying in my beer and telling this gray-haired, leathery old dude that I would give up my seat in hell to ride a Harley again.

He knew I was blind. He had to know, for two reasons. Number one: My seeing-eye brunette (Barbara) had been leading me through the bar for months. Number two: I always wore sunglasses in public. When people ask why I do this I answer, "Because the sun never sets on cool."

When we had finished the last set Barbara was packing the equipment and I was sitting at the bar when I felt a tap on my shoulder. A voice said, "Come on."

"What?" I said.

He said, "Come on, you wanted to ride, didn't you?"

I was good and loaded. I got up and followed him outside. I was hanging on to his arm so I assumed he knew of my blindness, because believe me when I tell you that if this old boy would have had the slightest suspicion that I was gay, I wouldn't be here to write this book.

"Miss Kitty," the neon nurse (bartender), must have overheard our conversation, for she immediately began to run up and down the bar yelling at the top of her lungs, "You can't let him do this."

By now everyone in the establishment knew what was going on. THE BLIND MAN WAS GONNA RIDE A HARLEY.

He stood beside the bike and said, "Get on."

I got on and received quick instructions— kick starter, clutch, gas, etc.

This time I was definitely shaking like a whore in church. I hadn't been on a motorcycle in twenty-five years, and it had been much longer since I had been at the controls. It felt good, but I was scared shitless.

By now Miss Kitty was hysterical. "Michael, please don't do this," she begged. Everyone was standing around in their drunken glory, urging me on. She ran to the stage where Barbara was packing our gear and said, "You've got to stop him." I'll always remember Barbara's reply as she casually stated over her shoulder, "He'll do nothing he can't handle."

I fired up the engine and sat there taking it all in. It was so "macho" with all that power between my legs. I wanted to roar down the street. I was filled with the motorcycle fantasies of my youth.

The concrete parking lot completely surrounded the building. I was ready to give it a try, but I am a survivor, and my instinct told me that it couldn't happen. There were a few too many obstacles, such as light poles, dumpsters, etc out there.

I had to gracefully remove myself from this situation, and Miss Kitty would be the unknowing catalyst. I said, "Okay, Miss Kitty, I'll ride bitch." (For those of you unfamiliar with biker slang, "bitch" is a polite term for passenger.)

I climbed on behind the old biker and we took off. It was February, and 2 a.m. as we roared through the night. I was wearing a tank top and quite comfortable. I was in a dreamland called "Southern California on a Harley."

After cruising a couple of miles he wheeled into a parking lot, put the bike in neutral, dismounted, and said, "There you go." It took a moment to register, but then I understood. He wanted me to drive.

I thought he was messin' with the kid, so I merely chuckled, but then I realized he wasn't joking. I said, "Man, you don't understand. All bullshit aside, I can't see."

For a moment there was total silence as he contemplated my exclamation. It dawned on me then that he was considering the possibility that he might be the one being taken for a ride, and being a veteran bullshitter himself, he was not about to let this happen.

As for "yours truly," I was acutely aware of the fact that I was out in the middle of nowhere with the big bad wolf, on the back of a Harley, in the wee hours of the morning, and I couldn't see shit. "I said, "Man, I'm serious, you don't want me to drive."

After what seemed like an eternity I finally convinced him that I couldn't see, and he climbed on the Sportster, and we returned to the club, where everyone was anxiously awaiting our arrival. As was customary we gathered inside for after hours complimentary drinks.

I wanted my old biker buddy to know I was straight with him, so I instructed Barbara and the gang to convince him beyond doubt, and they enthusiastically took up the challenge.

About an hour and several drinks later, over the noise of the crowd I heard my biker buddy exclaim, "Oh my God! Are you serious?" Reality was sinking in, for I believe he now understood the circumstances. This old gray-haired, pony-tailed, hard-core, Harley-rider had tried to talk a blind man into giving him the ride of his life.

The story, however, was far from over, for seldom do bikers have the occasion to tell tales of a blind man piloting their machine. A year passed and we once again returned to T's Roadhouse for another season of music and fun in the sun. Things hadn't changed much (same circus, same clowns), and I was right at the top of the heap. My old biker buddy was there, and he recalled our midnight ride vividly. He said, "Man, I couldn't believe that shit. I thought you were kiddin'. I got drunker that night than I'd been in years."

It was toward the end of our second season, and it seemed there were more bikers hanging out than usual. I had been singing, playing the guitar, and sweating for hours. It was "Miller Time." I was sitting at the bar relaxing, and I must admit I was feeling no pain when a voice said, "Come on."

There were four or five bikers, and I said, "What's up?"

They said, "Come on, you're gonna ride."

Of course I began to protest, reminding them of my eyesight, and they said, "Don't worry man, we have a plan." They were bikers and I was shit-faced, so what else could I do but stagger out the door with them?

Once outside they told me of their plan. "Pup" would position himself about 50 feet ahead of me while yelling at the top of his lungs to guide me. I would be flanked on my right and left by a Hell's Angel. While their intentions were well-meaning, they failed to understand that the roar of the Harley engines made it difficult to hear Pup's voice.

I was once again straddling Ponytail Terry's Sportster from the previous year, and he was riding "bitch."

I sat there revving the engine, and man, did it feel good. As I eased the clutch out and the bike began to move I came to a sudden realization. When riding a two-wheeler it is essential to have a reference point to balance yourself. If you don't believe this, try to ride a bicycle or motorcycle while wearing a blindfold.

Necessity being the mother of invention, I began to drag my feet to obtain a sense of balance. It worked, but I recommend wearing an old pair of shoes.

As the procession moved around the building I began to gain confidence. I was doing it. I was riding a Harley and I was blind. It was a blast. Everyone was yelling and cheering me on.

Over my shoulder I yelled at Ponytail Terry, "How far ahead of me is Pup?"

"About 75 feet," he replied.

I could stand it no longer. I revved the engine and popped the clutch. As I did so Ponytail Terry's feet flew up, and I nearly lost him.

As the engine roared and the tires squalled it was obvious that I would have to shut the machine down quickly or bad things would happen. I would experience the thrill of power and speed, no more than a few seconds, but for a brief moment I felt the thrill and excitement of youth.

When I brought the Harley to a stop I knew that I had come close to running "Pup" over.

I had calculated the distance quite well, for I had missed him by inches. He was standing to my immediate left and was so close to the bike I could have reached out and touched him. He said, "Jesus! Man, you almost ran over me."

We completed our ride around the building, and everyone was excited, especially me. They were patting me on the back and telling me what a great job I had done, and I was grinning like a butcher's dog; but not one person suggested another circle around the bar.

I was reminded of a time many years earlier when some of my buddies decided it might be fun to turn a blind man loose behind the wheel of a '58 Chevy in the middle of a snow-covered field. In both cases, however, their enthusiasm would abandon them as the adventure progressed, and to this day, I have had no request for a repeat performance.

At this time I must tell you of Ron, the proprietor of T's Roadhouse, for you see, he is a person who is fascinated by my blindness. Don't get me wrong, he's a great guy, but like so many people, he freaks out when he's around me. There are many who are uneasy about the reality of blindness.

This was obvious with Ron, because my blindness was always the main topic of discussion.

To Barbara he would say, "Why did you dress him in a pink shirt?" It became a standing source of humor. Finally it was the end of the season, and it was time for Michael to have some fun.

Somehow we found a pink t-shirt, and on the night of our last gig, it was eagerly worn. The trap was set and my buddy Ron eagerly took the bait. He staggered to the stage and said, "Mac, I love your pink shirt," and I answered in my usual way, "I'm not gonna fall for that b s, I'm blind, not stupid."

I could hardly contain my laughter for, as predicted, Ron became excited, saying, "No man, this time I'm not kidding." I said, "Give me a break."

He proceeded to gather witnesses, and bringing them to me, he would ask them to describe the color of my shirt. I was prepared for this. I said, "Yeah, you told them what to say."

It was so damned funny because, for the remainder of the night, Ron would repeatedly come to me and say, "I promise I'm not lying. You really do have a pink t-shirt on," and I would politely smile and say, "Bullshit!"

Finally, toward the end of the night, as Ron and his wife, Teresa, were leaving, I heard him say to Barbara, "You really should tell Mac the color of shirt he is wearing."

When Ron reads this book, as I am sure he will, he may possibly realize my awareness of the color of my attire. I hope I'm not being presumptuous, but I'm relatively certain he can read.

Several days passed, and we dropped by T's Roadhouse to have a cocktail and bid farewell to our friends. Oh yes, and also Ron. (Just kidding Ron, if you can read this.) It was closing time, and once again we were "shit-faced." Ron, being his usual fun-loving self, had another brilliant idea whereby they would be sufficiently entertained, and I'll give you three guesses as to who would be the star of his little show.

Ron had somehow procured an electric cart. You know the kind I refer to; they have the dubious distinction of being hotrods for old people in grocery stores, so he thought it would be hilarious to sit a blind man behind the wheel of one of these contraptions.

I seated myself behind the wheel and immediately began to have fun, and again, it was at Ron's expense. His first mistake was allowing himself to be in front of a vehicle which this blind man was driving, for I was determined to run him over. His second mistake was making noise, for in doing so, I could easily mark his location.

Words cannot describe the joy I felt as I chased Ron around his bar, for being a veteran musician; I found it difficult to acknowledge club owners as being human. (If you can read this, I love you Ron.)

Unfortunately, between Ron and myself there were many tables and chairs. I was reminded of bumper cars in an amusement park, and a blind hippie hillbilly musician was trying to flatten a club-owner clown.

For the next ten minutes I had the time of my life. There were few tables and chairs in the bar remaining upright. I was hot on Ron's tail, and he was yelling, "Okay, that's enough," and I was smiling and thinking, "I don't think so buddy."

I managed to bump him a few times, but somehow he avoided the wrath of the geriatric demon.

I gave up my quest to turn Ron into road kill, and as Miss Kitty tended to the business of reconstructing the bar, Ron and I sipped a tasty farewell beverage. Someday I plan to visit Cathedral City, and you can bet your pink t-shirt, Ron will be waiting.

It was also during our last season in the Palm Springs area when, while playing music at a place called The Saloon in Palm Springs, a very interesting event took place. Before I tell the story let me say I have entertained in practically every state in the Union, including Hawaii. I've rubbed elbows with the blue bloods at the country club in Palm Springs and slept on pool tables in the honky-tonks with the good old boys in Austin, Texas, but I can truthfully report to you that I have never feared for my personal safety nor felt such an acute sense of unease as I did in "The Saloon."

This place was as close to hell as you're going to get. Homeless people would wander in from the streets, and women would be on the dance floor with buck knifes strapped to their boots.

I was attempting to entertain these creatures to the best of my ability when a drunk staggered in and shouted in my direction, "I'll take that goddamned guitar from that blind son-of-a-bitch and show him how to play it." Mostly I am a very passive person, but this guy got my attention. I remember thinking, "You come up on this stage, baby, and you're gonna see a blind man come alive."

I found myself unable to play guitar or remember song lyrics, for I was formulating a plan of battle. If he stepped on my stage, the real show was about to begin. I'm not a bad ass, but the only thing worse than a blind man is a frightened blind man, especially this one.

After having completed several songs unscathed, my anxiety began to subside. I finished the set and had sat down to relax when I was given the details of the events unfolding outside.

It seems the bouncer's girlfriend, upon overhearing the insulting remarks directed toward me, promptly reported the incident to her man, who, in turn, proceeded to escort the idiot from the premises. After having done this the bouncer returned and told his friend what had happened. As fate would have it I had conversed with his friend earlier in the evening and must have made a favorable impression, for when he heard of his amigo being verbally abused, he immediately flew into a rage.

When speaking with him I could sense danger in this man, and he soon proved my suspicions warranted.

I was told he followed the guy outside and was on top of him. My new friend was beating the hell out of the troublemaker when the bouncer pulled him off and he was whisked away because someone had called the cops.

The cops arrived and brought the bad guy back inside so he could identify his attacker, who had long since fled the scene. This, however, was not the end of it, because some of the patrons began to harass the police, who were more than happy to provide three of them with free room and board.

While this was going on I was singing and playing my little heart out, oblivious of the fact that just outside, a few feet from me in an alley behind a dumpster, a good citizen would take it upon himself to defend my honor. It was not the first time this had happened nor would it be the last.

This story is one of my favorites. In 2000, around the time our great Republican president, George Herbert Walker Blankety Bush, was unfairly elected, Barbara and I were in Bullhead City, Arizona, on the Colorado River. If you want to gamble you must venture across the river to Laughlin, Nevada, where this particular sin just happens to be legal, as declared by the good citizens of that great state.

One night we were in a casino playing the nickel slot machines. It was around three a.m., and I was sitting at the bar after drinking copious amounts of Jack Daniels. Barbara was sitting to my right. She stated that she was going to the restroom, leaving me to ponder my drunken stupor.

She soon returned, and as I sat there, I casually placed my hand upon her back and began to gently massage.

As I gently performed this act of affection, I noticed that something was terribly wrong. The back I was caressing felt four feet wide. Just as I came to my senses and lifted my hand from this massive body, a deep, husky voice said, "Excuse me sir. Would you please remove your hand from my back?"

I became instantly sober. I began to sweat and I'm sure my pulse rate tripled. My mind was racing 90 miles an hour. I sat in stunned silence.

As my intellect slowly returned I began to understand what had happened.

I was in a casino, not in a local bar down the street. Having been born and raised in the buckle of the Bible belt, casinos were a new experience for me. Perched on the bar in front of the seat to my immediate right was a video poker game patiently waiting for a big bruiser to sit down and empty his pockets into it.

I don't know how long I sat there. I was in shock. Barbara had returned and was sitting to my left. I kept my hands on the bar and, facing forward, called, "Barbara?" I cannot begin to describe how relieved I was when I heard her voice.

I must have been giving off some serious vibes because she immediately wanted to know if I was feeling all right. I just wanted to get the hell out of there.

As we were leaving I kept asking her if we were being followed. Not until we were safely in our vehicle and returning to Bullhead City did I relay my unusual story to her. Bless her little heart. She laughed so hard it was necessary to pull off the road and park until she regained composure.

About a week later, thinking mostly of complimentary drinks, I was lured into the casino once again. By this time I had become familiar with the bartender. I asked if he would guide me to the little boy's room as I had to beat the piss out of my best friend. He obliged, and I was returned once again to my seat.

I revisited the casino a few nights later and was shocked to learn that my neon nurse had nearly lost his job because he had helped his blind buddy to the rest room.

Upon reviewing the security tapes the next day, it seems the young security officers were quite perplexed at the sight of a man wearing sunglasses after dark, with hair down to his ass, being led into the men's room by the bartender. Imagine that.

As there were no cameras in the privy they suspected a drug deal. Man, these kids were street-wise.

That night, the more drinks I consumed the more incensed I became. By God! In the morning I would call my lawyer, and it would be litigation city.

Finally, after many glasses of courage, I decided on instant satisfaction. To hell with lawyers and court rooms! I stood and raised my middle finger.

With a broad smile I made a 360 degree turn so the cameras would miss nothing. That was totally out of character for me, but man, it felt great.

I expected to be escorted from the casino at any moment, but it didn't happen. The security boys must have been watching porno flicks on the other monitor.

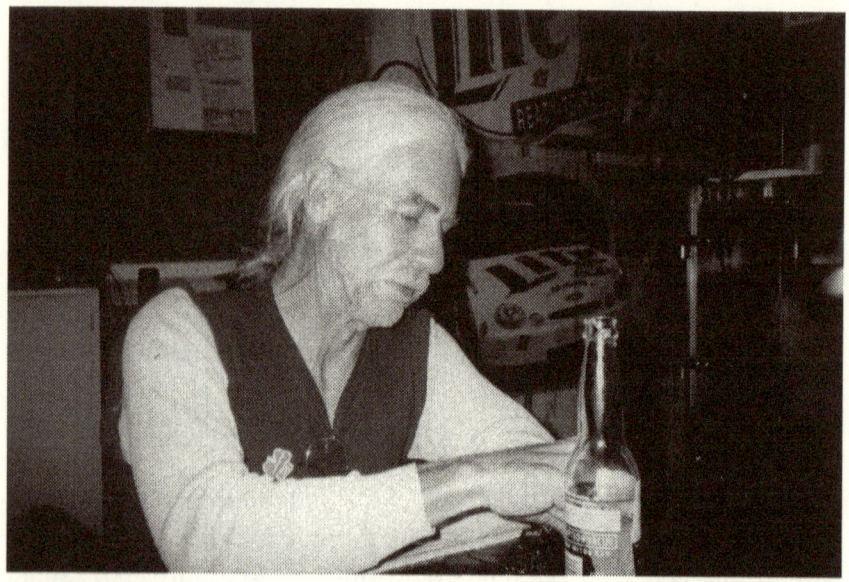

Ponytail Terry

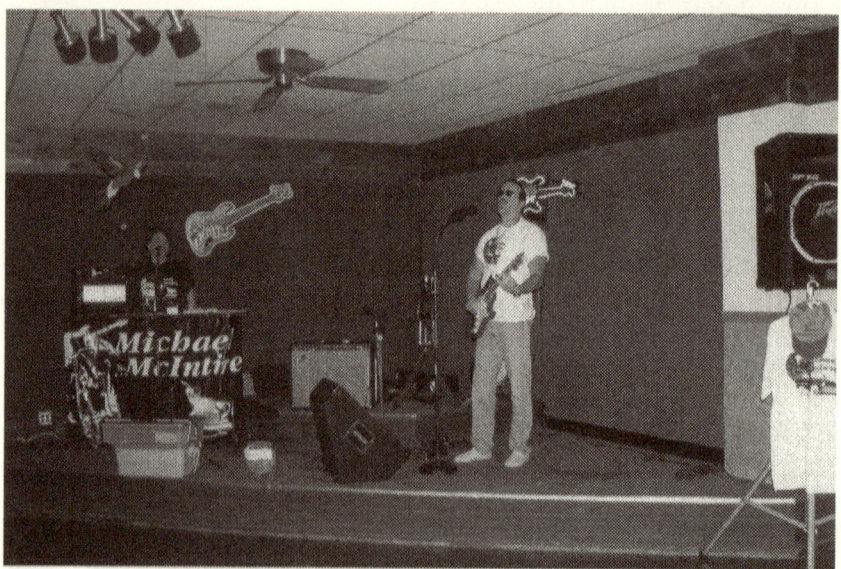

Michael and Barbara Hoskin (on the road) at a gig

Chapter 10
More Crazy Stories

In this chapter I shall throw chronology to the wind and write what comes to mind. For instance, as I write this book the blind adventure continues. The Blind Fairy has not forsaken me because yesterday, June 2, 2004, I had another close call.

Workmen were doing repairs on my screened-in deck at the rear of my home. The roof had been leaking and they were trying to locate the problem, so with coffee cup in hand, I would lend my expertise. I opened the screen door and stepped outside, only to find myself where I have been many times in my life. Once again I had stepped into space. My brain blew a fuse. What the hell was going on? Why was the top step no longer where it was supposed to be?

My right leg went through the space where the step should have been, finally touching the ground about three feet down. My left leg, however, was at the upper level. To give you an idea of my situation, my left knee was almost to my chin.

Luckily my right hand was clasping the cedar post of the door frame. With the thumb and forefinger of my right hand I was also holding the coffee cup. This meant that I was holding the weight of my 190 pound body with three fingers.

I managed to pull myself from the opening with minor injuries. This morning my lower back is a little stiff, and those three fingers on my right hand are somewhat swollen, but I realize it could have been much worse.

The workmen had removed the top step to make adjustments, but they had not taken the time to inform me of this. Oh well, just another day in the life of a blind man.

It was 1973 and the square in downtown Springfield had recently been renovated. In the middle of the square was a large decorative water fountain just begging for mischief. Another of my so-called friends, David Pearson, and I had just closed down a bar and were staggering home. Dave was playing the role of intoxicated human guide dog. Having had no training for this job, he was doing remarkably well.

Let me describe the scene for you. We're just a couple of young guys out sowing our wild oats at two a.m. I'm twenty-three and Dave is nineteen. We both have long hair; mine reached the middle of my back. I am clasping Dave's arm as we stagger across the empty square. It must have been a sight to behold.

I could hear the fountain as we approached. By now you've probably noticed that throughout my life, I seem to attract people with the same sordid sense of humor as I myself possess.

When Dave said, "Okay, step up and then about five steps in front of you, take another step," I knew what was coming, but I thought to myself, "I'm just in the mood to play along."

I yelled with surprise as I splashed into the water. Assuming he had sufficiently fooled the blind boy, my buddy Dave was beside himself. We were laughing our asses off and having a good ole time. How nice of the city to provide us with our very own play pool.

When Dave extended his hand to assist me as I exited the fountain, I naturally insisted he join me. It seemed to take forever to remove ourselves from the fountain, because the slime in the bottom made it nearly impossible to stand upright. I would help him to his feet only to once again take my seat. Finally we struggled to the ledge, and as we made our exit I heard a deep, authoritative voice say, "What do you boys think you're doing?" It was Mr. Policeman, and he was not enjoying the party.

We removed ourselves from the water and stood grinning and dripping before the constable. He was not amused. After checking our soggy identification he asked why we were in his fountain.

As I had done, and was destined to do many times in my life, I began to explain my unique situation to this law enforcement officer who was very close to our age. I told him I was legally blind, and my friend was helping me across the square when he was overcome with an uncontrollable urge to walk me into the fountain. I thought this would placate the cop and he would merely shrug and we could be on our way, but to my surprise, he freaked out.

"I don't think that's funny," he exclaimed. "What kind of a friend would walk you into the fountain like that?" Hell! He was ready to escort my old buddy Dave to jail.

It took all my persuasive skills to keep this from happening. About 30 minutes later he let us go, and I've kicked myself in the ass a thousand times for not doing things differently.

What a difference thirty years can make. In the same situation today I would keep my mouth shut, and let nature run its course. Once again we were going to have some fun with the blind guy, and I was okay with that, but I was given a perfect opportunity to turn the tables. Can you imagine? If the cop had thrown Dave in jail I would still be laughing.

By now you may have concluded that my friends were poorly chosen if they would play such pranks as guiding me into a water fountain, but this next story may help redeem their character. Throughout my life the Blind Fairy had plenty of help, for I was blessed with many thoughtful and protective buddies, some of whom would have given their life for me.

One night in 1973, my friend Michael Libertus, whom I have mentioned several times in this book, and I were returning from a party near campus in Springfield when the serpent of danger reared its ugly head.

We were driving from the apartment complex where the party had been held when we were flagged down by a guy who promptly presented himself at my window on the passenger side. He said, "Are you wearing green wire-rim glasses?"

I was incredulous. When I recovered from this off the wall and idiotic question, I responded, "Yes."

Suddenly all hell broke loose. I was pulled toward the driver's side with great force. At the same instant I heard a loud bang. Later I was told this sound was a fist striking the inside of the vehicle, missing my head by inches.

Fortunately, having been schooled in martial arts, Michael instinctively reacted with lightning speed and pulled me from harm's way.

We got the hell out of there, but our surprise would soon turn to anger, and by the time we got home we were furious.

Having been viciously attacked without provocation, we wanted to know the reason, so a posse was hastily formed. By God, if they wanted to dance, we would provide the music.

Among those in the posse was my friend Dave Pearson. You may remember Dave as being the person instigating the Saturday night bath in the city water fountain. There was also Leroy, a black dude from Kansas City.

The posse parked in front of the party house, got out, and walked in. Our social grace must have been lacking, for we forgot to knock. It didn't take long to locate my attacker. He was stretched out on a couch in the living room.

Imagine his surprise when, upon opening his eyes, he found himself surrounded by a group of young men, and they were not smiling.

He failed to recognize us at the onset of this encounter, but we were more than happy to help refresh his memory.

I couldn't see what was going on, but by this time I was fired up and ready to go. I demanded an explanation. He said someone had told him I was a narcotics agent. This really got me going, for such a rumor would be a sure death sentence.

Dave and Leroy were ready to open up a can of whip-ass. It was all I could do to hold them off, and to this day I don't know why I did.

When the idiot spoke I could detect fear in his voice. He was on his own, for the other people in the house had mysteriously vanished.

I was an inexperienced youth of twenty-three, but I knew this was a serious situation. I stepped forward and, standing directly in front of him as he sat on the couch, told him I was not now, nor had I ever been, a narc. I explained the danger of such rumors, and how he should get his facts straight before attacking total strangers. Finally I said, "We're leaving, but if I hear one word from anyone about this we'll be back."

We had to practically drag Dave and Leroy out the door.

In 1974 my life-long buddies Michael Libertus and Greg Parker along with yours truly opened a bar in Springfield. Located on Commercial at Campbell, it was called The Joint. Those were rockin' times. The place was packed every weekend, the booze flowed, and there were so many young, beautiful hippie chicks I was like a kid in a candy store.

After about three months I had my fill of the business end of it, so I told my partners they could have my share of the bar if they would waive the cover charge and provide all the booze I could drink free of charge.

They agreed and I became the bar mascot. I was there every night checkin' out the ladies and catchin' a buzz.

Man, I thought I was Mr. Cool, being 6 feet -2 inches with hair to my waist. I would stand at the bar and wait for my prey just like a spider patiently waiting for a fly.

I was standing at the bar sipping a beer one night when the bouncer said, "Mac, you'd better move away because a guy has a gun and I think there's gonna be trouble."

Well, needless to say, he didn't have to repeat himself. I moved away. I began to walk toward the nearest lighted area, which happened to be the foosball table. As I approached, people began to scramble away, except for one guy. My vision was much better in those days, and I could see his face under the light.

He was looking right at me as he stepped back. If I could have seen his face clearly, I'm sure I would have recognized that DON'T MESS WITH ME look on his face, but oblivious to what was going on, I kept walking.

Suddenly I saw something. It was a bright, metallic reflection, and it moved fast. There was a commotion, and I could hear people scuffling.

The incident took about two seconds to play itself out. Hell, I didn't know what was going on. By the time it was over I was but six feet from the guy.

I was later told that the bouncer had asked the guy to leave and he refused, saying he had a gun. When the guy saw the bouncer talking to me and then saw me move in his direction he must have assumed I was Billy bad-ass, and I planned to make him eat that chrome-plated pistol.

I now knew why he had that freaked-out look on his face as he stepped back. The poor guy had no way of knowing I couldn't see, so I'll bet he thought I was one bad cat. He drew down on me as, just like Steve McQueen, I casually walked in his direction. In a flash he was disarmed by several of my associates and promptly escorted to the door. Thanks again, Blind Fairy.

Here's one you can appreciate. After a night at The Joint my partners, some friends, and I decided to party at our house. As we entered the door we noticed four or five rolled up newspapers on the porch. My dear friend Greg Parker decided it would be loads of fun to turn out the lights and have a good old fashioned paper fight with the blind man. Yep, here we go again, but it's all in fun. Right?

At first I was apprehensive, but when they turned the lights off, I felt quite comfortable, knowing there was a room full of blind people. Excuse me; they were drunk blind people, or blind drunks. Take your pick.

Within seconds I had control of the situation, and I would show no mercy. It was so easy because all I had to do was listen for the sound of breathing. I would calculate the exact location of the sound, then very quietly raise the rolled paper and, grasping it with both hands, bring it down on the head of my dear friends using every ounce of strength I possessed.

I smile as I write this. Oh, such fond memories. Once again, they were going to have some fun at my expense, but they just didn't realize one very important point. When my fun-loving, sighted friends turned the lights off, they entered my world.

It wasn't long before my friend Dan Reese flipped the lights on and stated, "I've had enough."

I remained unscathed, and I'll bet that was the shortest paper fight in history.

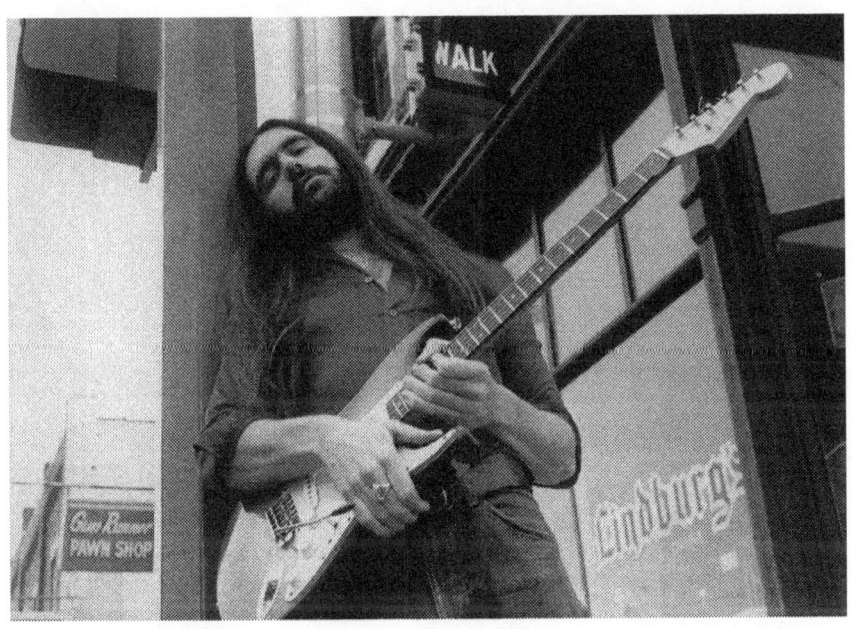

Michael outside of Linburg's, formally "The Joint,"
of which he was part owner in 1974.
(Photo taken by Donna 'Pokie' Alrutz)

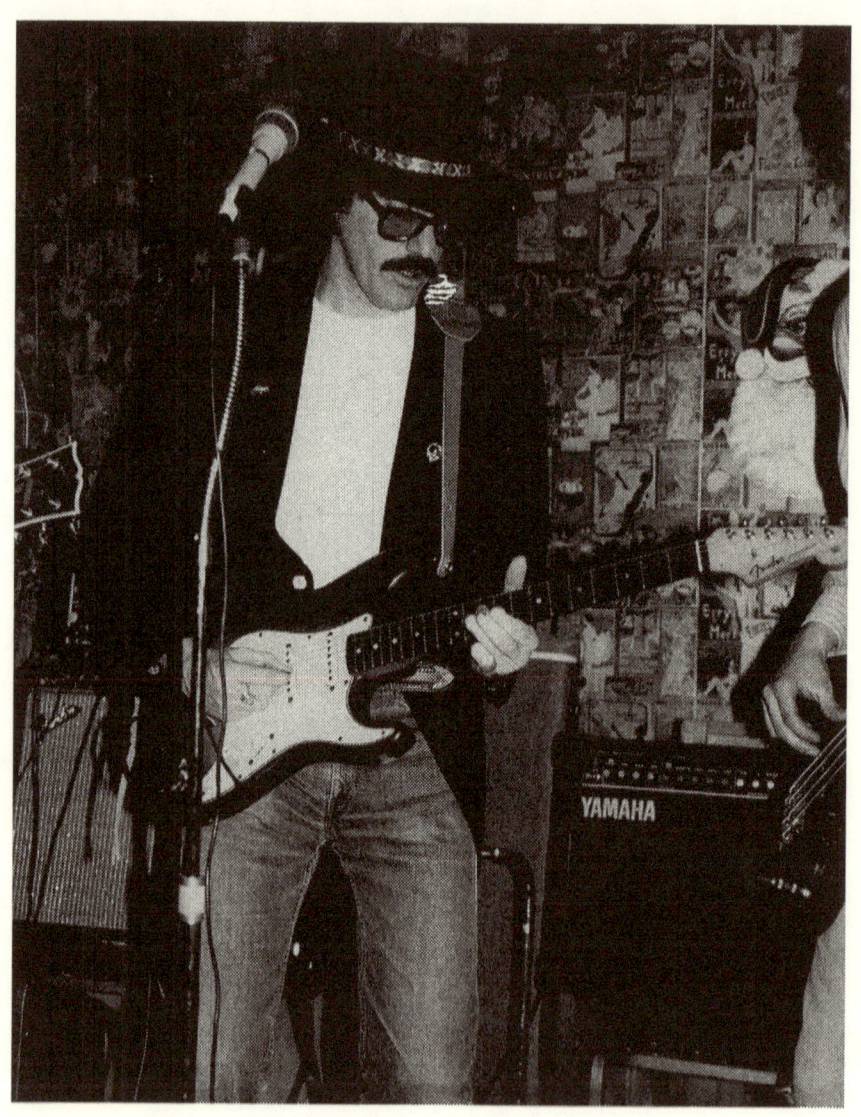

The Electric Man

Chapter 11
Danger Is My Music

Mom, if you suffer from anxiety about your son or daughter becoming a rock'n'roll musician, urge them to read this chapter, as it could possibly effect their decision.

Around 1985 I was playing music three nights a week at a local dive in Springfield, Missouri. It was known as The Dugout, but we appropriately named it The Slugout, for reasons which will soon become obvious.

The joint was usually filled to capacity on a nightly basis, but around 10 p.m. there would be a brawl and most of the customers would promptly make their exit. If it had not been for the almighty dollar I can assure you that Michael McIntire would have done the same.

One night I was singing and daydreaming simultaneously. This is common when you have been singing the song hundreds of times through the years.

My dream was interrupted when, from the lighted area around the pool table, I saw a woman grasping billiard balls and vigorously hurling them at someone. If you've held a billiard ball in your hand you know the damage this would cause to a human skull.

I turned to the drummer and cried, "If those balls land on stage I'm out of here."

Now it was well known that I had poor eyesight, and something about my excitement and fear made the drummer laugh so hard he could no longer play. We were forced to take a break.

Several weeks later while playing music at the same bar, I found myself in a most bizarre situation. We had just finished a set, and as I was being led from the stage my foot struck something and I nearly fell. Inquiring of this, I was informed it was a human body.

It seems that while I was pouring my heart out to the audience, an altercation had ensued just a few feet from where I was standing. Man, talk about getting into your music!

I was told that some idiot busted another idiot over the head with a cue stick, causing him to take a power nap at my feet.

That in itself speaks volumes, for I had an excuse. I couldn't see. The poor bastard could have passed on, and it would have gone unnoticed.

One time in the early 90s my band The Blues Project had returned to Springfield from a gig in Hot Springs, Arkansas. We had driven the band members home with the exception of the drummer, Dave Peterson, who was passed out in the back seat.

My lady, Debbie Hediger, was the designated wheel woman. When we finally arrived at Dave's house it was around 3 a.m. Debbie wanted to let him sleep it off in the van, but I was determined to take him home, for I didn't want to deal with it the next day.

I opened the side door and tried to wake him, but he didn't respond. I grasped him by the ankles and proceeded to drag him from the vehicle, thinking this would revive him, but to no avail.

After what seemed to take forever we were approaching the entrance to his house, when suddenly his carcass came to life.

He became quite belligerent. He began to shove me. I couldn't believe the strength this man possessed. I weighed about 180 pounds, and he was pushing me around as if I were a child.

Acutely aware of my blindness, Debbie's maternal instincts must have kicked in, for she was there in an instant. She tried to place her coat between us to deter his onslaught.

He said, "You get out of here, bitch." Debbie began to sob. She took me by the arm, and we began a hasty retreat toward the van. He was close behind, screaming obscenities as we closed and locked the doors. While we were getting the hell out of Dodge he hurled a half-filled beer can at us as a going away gift.

Not until we had driven several blocks did I learn the details of Dave Peterson's violent actions. When Debbie tossed the coat between us she was not only attacked verbally, but physically as well.

The sorry excuse for a human being struck Debbie in the face with his fist, breaking her glasses. Understandably she was shaken to the point of hardly being able to drive.

As for me, I was furious—in fact, my head was spinning. By nature, I'm not an impulsive person. I prefer to formulate a plan, covering my ass as I go. The Chinese have a saying: "Revenge is a dish best served cold."

I told Debbie to say the word and I would form a posse, and Dave Peterson would wish to God he'd never been born.

She just wanted to let it go, and I understood. Her son Danny had a temper, and if he knew what had taken place, Dave Peterson had better give his heart to God, because the rest of him would belong to Danny.

I would later learn of Dave Peterson's drug problem and the fact that he was on parole. Not surprisingly, he broke parole and was returned to the slammer, where hopefully, he resides to this day.

In 1980 I happened to be living in Eminence, Missouri, where my beautiful twin daughters were conceived. I had met their mother, Bebe Bryant, in Fort Collins, Colorado, while playing music on the road with Roger Sanders.

Bebe and I moved to the hills to take a break from the hustle and bustle of city life. She is an excellent vocalist. She is featured on my album, *Runnin' Wild*.

Having no intention of totally abandoning the life of a musician, we would occasionally get together with our friends and drive to a small town in Missouri and wow them with our music.

On one such occasion we found ourselves in Iberia, Missouri, a large metropolis with a population of roughly five-hundred hillbillies.

We were in the middle of our fourth set when I heard a familiar sound. If you've been in a bar when a fight breaks out you know what I'm talking about. It sounds like a tornado, hurricane, and a domestic disturbance all happening at the same time.

When the fun began Bebe took my arm (maternal instinct), and we dashed for cover. Upon reaching a relatively safe position, I immediately became aware of the fact that I had left my guitar behind, and my precious baby was but a few feet from a good old boy disaster.

It must have been one hell of a sight, for Bebe had dragged me from the stage and possible danger. Now I was dragging her toward the stage as she was trying to keep me from getting hillbilly killed. Nothing would keep me from my baby. It was a 1962 Fender Stratocaster I had purchased from Randy Thomas for two-hundred and fifty dollars, and by God I was going back for it.

Fortunately, by the time I had reached the stage, things were under control.

The Blind Fairy must have intervened once again, for I couldn't see a damned thing. I was navigating by sound, instinct, fear, and anger.

When it was over I was told that earlier in the evening our bass player, Jim Wyrick, had a disagreement with the bouncer. Allow me to translate. He shot his mouth off at the wrong guy.

We were in the middle of a song when the bouncer approached the stage, grabbed the bass player by the shirt, and yanked him off stage and onto the floor. He was standing next to me, and—guess what?—once again, Michael was totally unaware of what was going on.

Both men would weigh between 230 and 250 pounds. They were separated, and needless to say, the show was over, folks.

There were rumblings by the natives when we packed to leave, and I'll never forget the terrible sound of the rocks striking our car, as we made our escape.

Again I would find myself in a dangerous position in Virginia City, Nevada, while Barbara Hoskin and I were touring the West in 2001.

We had finished our gig and were invited to sit in with Will and Sheri Rose, who were playing Fly's Silver Dollar Saloon.

The place was packed. If you had become intoxicated to the point of passing out, you wouldn't have had to worry about hitting the floor because the mass of bodies would have given ample support.

Upon arrival, some idiot tried to remove my hat from my head. I am happy to report this endeavor to be unsuccessful. When you have spent most of your life in saloons you learn to sense danger, and I knew this was a portent of things to come.

Several hours and several drinks later I was on stage with the band. We were in the middle of a song when I was struck hard in the face. I stumbled backward as I tried to protect my guitar. My hat, which still bares the scars of the encounter, was knocked from my head. My glasses also parted from my face.

Talk about getting one's attention. In an instant I had my guitar off and was ready for action. There was only one problem. I couldn't see the action.

My mouth was numb where the microphone had smashed into it. Pain will certainly increase the flow of adrenalin.

I was confused, because the familiar sound of a brawl was not there. I was soon given a reason for this.

I discovered, to my astonishment, that the clown who had earlier tried to steal my hat from me had tried to steal the wrong man's wife and received his just reward.

The psychotic bastard was struck a beautiful, solid blow to the face, which sent him flying in this blind hippie hillbilly's direction.

When the clown got what he deserved he was around twenty-five feet from where I stood, but the force of the blow sent him reeling. He covered the distance without regaining his balance and collided with yours truly.

He had been knocked out, and I would later discover he had received a concussion. I'm certain it wasn't the first time he had been knocked on his ass, and it wouldn't be the last.

Once again I found myself with an idiot napping at my feet, and as I stood listening to the siren of the ambulance I remember thinking to myself, "Do you really want to be a musician?"

I should send a copy of this book to my congressman as it would definitely serve as an argument for laws to be passed pertaining to hazard pay for musicians. Yeah, right!

Speaking of hazardous, a few months ago (2004) I acted on a fantasy I've had for years. I've always wanted to dance on the bar. What's the big deal? Right? I suggest you try this blindfolded, and you will soon become educated.

I was seated in Buck and Billy's, a local bar not far from my home, when I was overcome by an irresistible urge to climb up there and strut my stuff.

I stood up and, grasping the edge, leaped upon the bar in a single bound.

The number one rule if you are blind is, NEVER ASSUME ANYTHING. People were always dancing on the bar, much to the owner's chagrin, but I didn't know they were midgets.

I'm around 6 feet, 2 inches, and when I stood up I soon became painfully aware of the distance between the bar and the ceiling, and I can testify it is much less than my height.

Man, it was the Fourth of July. I saw every color in the rainbow. I somehow regained composure and made my way down to the relative safety of the bar stool.

My fantasy will become reality. Someday I will dance on the bar, but you can rest assured I will take the proper measurements.

Around 1995 Debbie Hediger and I were playing a gig for the AmVets on West Sunshine in Springfield, Missouri. We were playing the last set of the night when, in the middle of a song, something hit me at the knees. It felt like a ton of bricks and could have easily broken my legs.

Naturally, I didn't see this coming, and it's easy to imagine my shock and anger as I tried to figure out what the hell was going on.

Ironically, the lady who had fallen into me was Barbara Hoskin. Her name has been mentioned periodically throughout this book. As fate would have it we would live together for six years and travel the West playing music, but at the time we hardly knew each other.

Debbie and I would have the horrible misfortune a few months later of being hit head-on by a drunk driver in Springfield, at which time my partner and loving companion of eight years and six months would lose her life.

A short time after Barbara and I began sharing our lives together, she explained to me what had happened. She said her boyfriend at the time, Rocky Thomas, was spinning her while dancing and released her hand, sending her flying in my direction.

Please allow this writer to indulge himself in a moment of philosophy. We like to imagine ourselves to be in control of our lives, but this is utter nonsense. In other words, we can set our sails, but who can tell which way the wind will blow?

I would have another close call in 1982. We were returning to our home in Fort Collins from a gig in Estes Park, Colorado. If you've driven down Poudre Canyon in the Rocky Mountains you know what a treacherous drive this can be, especially at 3 a.m. when you're tired and buzzed out.

We were in our bass player Matt Powellson's Volkswagen. Matt, having relinquished the wheel due to a disagreement with tequila, was in the back seat.

Suddenly Matt had the urge to purge, and we offered no resistance when he ordered us to pull over. I was in the front passenger seat, and when the car stopped I got out and opened the door for his exit, for understandably we wanted him out of the car as soon as humanly possible.

Instantly, as Matt stepped from the car I heard sounds I will never forget. For one brief moment I was transported back in time, hunting coons at night in the Ozark Mountains as a teenager.

I heard grunts, falling rocks, tree limbs snapping, and the thumping sound of something heavy as it connected with the ground. There was also the sound of water running, and in the distance below someone was moaning.

Being my usual smartass self, I stuck my head in the window of the car and said calmly, "I think we've lost him." Soon we devised an ingenious method of extraction. We formed a human chain, and after an exhaustive effort our bass player was rescued.

Miraculously, Matt was unscathed. As I recall, he sounded pretty relaxed as he went crashing down the mountain. If he had reached the stream it could have been fatal, because the water is extremely cold. Fortunately, Matt would live to play bass guitar on *my album, "Runnin Wild*.

There was a distance of only three feet from the vehicle to oblivion. This time my blindness would save me. As I exited the car I instinctively didn't let go of the door. Had I stepped away from the car, this story may have had a very tragic outcome. Thank you, Blind Fairy.

Around the time my twin daughters were born I had another harrowing experience in the same canyon. We were returning from a gig in Estes Park when one of our tires blew. What a place to have a blowout! If you left the road while driving down that canyon, chances are you would never be found.

Fortunately, Bebe managed to safely bring the car to a halt. Under different circumstances a flat tire would be no big deal, but when I took stock of my situation I slumped in my seat, for I knew I was in big trouble.

There were five of us in the car, and I was the only male. The passengers included my mother, two aunts, Bebe, and me.

To make matters worse, I had been drinking copious amounts of tequila, and it's as I always say, "The only thing worse than a blind man is a drunk blind man."

We were in a station wagon loaded with music equipment and with a malfunctioning tailgate that had, for the last few weeks, refused to open. On that fateful night I paid a high price for procrastination.

The spare tire was located in a compartment beneath the area where hundreds of pounds of music equipment patiently waited to be unloaded.

Man, talk about a buzz killer! Within a short time I was sober as a judge. Everything had to be unloaded from the rear passenger doors. When we finally removed the spare tire from the vehicle I remember standing there and thinking to myself, "What now?"

I was thirty years on this planet, and somehow the experience of changing a tire had escaped me. I had seen it done many times, however, so by remembering what I had observed, and with the women acting as my eyes, we set to work.

Of course it was slow going, but in about an hour we were on the road again, as Willie says. I took two things from this. Number one: If something is broken, fix it, and number two: I could change a flat tire with a blindfold on.

Another Wild West adventure happened on the road between Laramie, Wyoming, and Fort Collins, Colorado, while returning from making music in Saratoga Springs, Wyoming.

It was a bright, sunny day, and we were on a flat two lane highway. My friend Jude Barnum was driving her 1956 Ford pick-up truck.

We were cruising along about 65 mph, which seemed like 100 in that old tin can. Looking up from my nap I happened to notice we were headed out across the prairie, so I reacted as anyone would. I screamed, "What the hell are you doing?"

I now know this was not the correct response, because she also reacted as anyone would. She over-corrected, and the fun began.

Jerking the wheel to the left brought us back to the highway, but by this time we were broadside and in the left lane. When she jerked the wheel to the right again, that was all she wrote.

That old top-heavy truck started rolling down the highway like a toy being kicked down the sidewalk.

I remember the sensation of the truck leaving the ground during the first two rolls, and after each roll I was so grateful to be living.

When it finally came to a stop the vehicle was on its side. Everything was dark. It was like being in a cavern. My glasses were gone, and I lay crumpled on the driver's side, which was now the floorboard.

I could smell gasoline and I heard hissing sounds, so I got the hell out of there. In one motion I popped the passenger door open, grabbed the running board, executed a perfect summersault, and hit the ground running.

During this time I could hear Jude crying in the distance. I ran toward this sound, and upon reaching her I found she had been thrown from the truck, and the truck had rolled over her.

People had arrived to lend a hand, so when I saw a bone in her leg sticking out about two inches I told her I was going to look for my guitar.

My guitar had been thrown out, and it was still in the case. We were both in working order. It was unbelievable, for the truck had rolled about six times. My hair was to my waist at the time, and the guy behind us said all he could see was arms, legs, and hair.

I played a gig the next night in Fort Collins, but I was sore from one end of my poor body to the other. I would also be plagued with nightmares for a few months, and my friend Jude walks with a cane to this day.

As I have written in this chapter, many unforgettable events have taken place during forty years of traveling the country playing music, but none could match the horror of the event which took place in Springfield, Missouri, at 1:35 a.m. on the night of October 15, 1995.

My lady Debbie Hediger and I were returning from a gig. While preparing to execute a left turn off Kansas Expressway onto Grant Street we were hit by a drunk driver. An officer told me he was traveling between 100 and 130 mph.

The Corvette was airborne when it struck our van precisely where Debbie was seated. Both vehicles were destroyed by fire, and I was miraculously pulled from the van.

I suffered fourteen fractures and am now the proud owner of a titanium plate in my upper jaw plus a titanium rod from my right elbow to my shoulder. My upper jaw was broken in eight places, and my lower jaw was broken in two places. My left hip was broken, and I had a collapsed lung, along with three broken ribs. Other than that, Mrs. Lincoln, how did you like the play?

I had to learn to play the guitar all over again, and it took three years to return to normal. That is to say, as close to normal as Michael McIntire could possibly be.

My lady and partner in life and music of more than eight years didn't make it.

Nothing before or since has had such a profound effect upon my life and music. I was transformed emotionally because of this living nightmare. When I play my guitar or sing, it's from the heart. I give it everything I've got. She is with me always. She was my biggest fan, and I shall always miss her humor and wit.

For over thirty years my mother would spend sleepless nights wondering if I safely arrived home after a gig. She finally received the dreaded call. Once, during a visit to the hospital, she said, "Surely, you're not going to keep playing music."

To discontinue my career in music is to stop living, and I know Debbie would want me to keep on rockin'.

Concerned parents can relax, for only a small minority of musicians actually sticks with it.

In my case it has not only been a passion but a lifestyle.

I wrote this description of the wreck, which took place October 15, 1995, to be given to the news media.

The Long Ride Home

By Michael McIntire
Springfield, Missouri – 1995

We were riding along just casually talking after a long weekend of playing music. We were exhausted. We had played Friday night in Shell Knob and Saturday night in Springfield. We had worked our second night and were on our way home. Debbie was Southbound on Kansas and was preparing to make a left turn on Grand. We were just a few minutes from home. She had put the turn signal on and was slowing down. The van was running about 30 miles per hour.

There were no headlights, no screaming tires, nothing to prepare us for what was to happen next.

I believe that time slows down because your mind accelerates. The first thought I remember having was; "My God they have finally hit us." Then I thought it might have been a train that hit us, but I knew this was not possible since there were no railroad tracks in the area. When the noise finally subsided my six foot and one-half inch frame occupied a small space in the floor board.

I found it hard to believe that I was still alive. Instinctively I knew Debbie and I should get out of the van immediately. I remember calling Debbie's name many times but there was no answer. I was like a small child trying to speak. I was unaware that my teeth were hanging out of the side of my face, my upper jaw was broken in eight places, my lower jaw in one place, my sinuses were crushed and that my nose was broken.

When I finally repositioned myself in the passenger seat I immediately tried to unlock the door. Unaware that my right arm was crushed at the biceps and was attached to my body only by a piece of skin. I started to reach with my left hand to open the door when suddenly I heard a voice say "Come on man." By this time a small crowd of about 15 to 20 people had congregated and were gazing in horror at the burning vehicles. I can understand why a person would not want to risk his or her life to save a busted up, blind musician trying to grope his way out of a burning van, but I am certainly forever grateful that the brave Mr. Duane Brainard was in that crowd.

He pulled me from the van and I hit the ground like a sack a potatoes. I was a rag doll. Along with my other injuries I had a broken hip, three broken ribs with a collapsed lung, and cuts and bruises from one end of my body to the other. Duane grabbed my belt in back and my collar at the back of my neck and began to drag me away from the van before it exploded. People rushed to help Duane drag my body along the ground. I was in shock, I felt no pain. The only time that I recall experiencing pain was when one of the people helping Duane took my arm that was hanging by skin and tried to drag me. Needless to say, he soon found another approach.

During this time I repeatedly told them that Debbie was in the van and that they needed to get her out. I would not let my mind think the worst. I thought, "I am alive so she must be alive." When they finally stopped dragging me someone covered me with a coat. A woman took my hand and was trying to comfort me. I now know what it feels like to die because I could feel the life slipping away from me. I was gasping for air. I told my angel of mercy that the ambulance had better get here soon. It finally arrived, but it seemed like an eternity. I was conscious the whole time, even in the emergency room. I kept begging for information about Debbie but I knew the truth. Finally, a nurse told me that Debbie was no longer with me. At first life meant nothing to me. It was when my mother walked into the emergency room and I saw the fear and pain and concern in her eyes that only a mother could have that I knew I should at least continue on for the sake of my loved ones.

It has been almost two years since the morning of October 15, 1995. I am much stronger now but the person I once was no longer exists. He is gone forever.

When Joe Willis Wright made the decision to get behind the wheel of the Corvette and put the pedal to the floor board and run between 100 and 130 miles per hour on a city street while blasted out of his mind, he could never know that the horrible events that would be set in motion would effect the lives of hundreds of people from out of state as well as locally.

Our roads are turning into a war zone and if we do not fight back we will continue to lose our loved ones because of those idiots behind the wheel who make the wrong choices.

I will never know why Debbie was taken and I was spared. I do know that she was a good person and that she touched many lives. My life was blessed just for having known and loved her, and as long as Michael McIntire is alive she will not be forgotten nor will her death be in vain.

Michael McIntire

(NOTE: From <u>http://blind-cat.com</u> -- To learn more about this event as it was reported in the news, see the Scrapbook segment of the Photo Gallery.

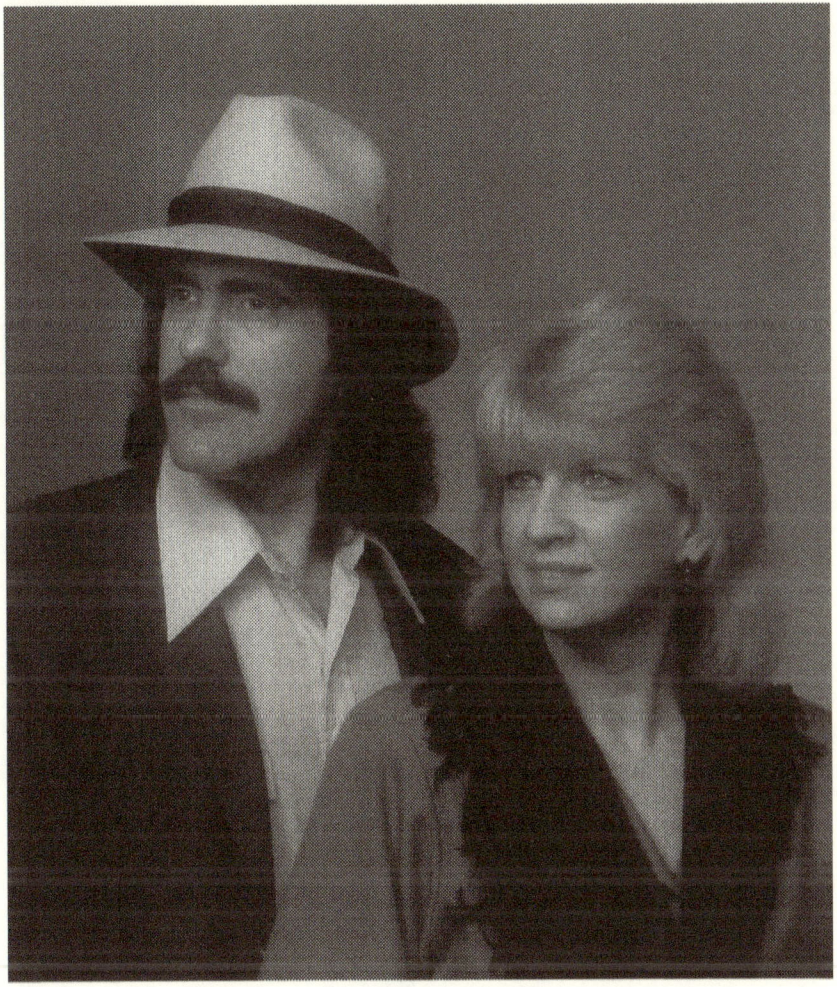

Michael and Debbie Hediger in 1989

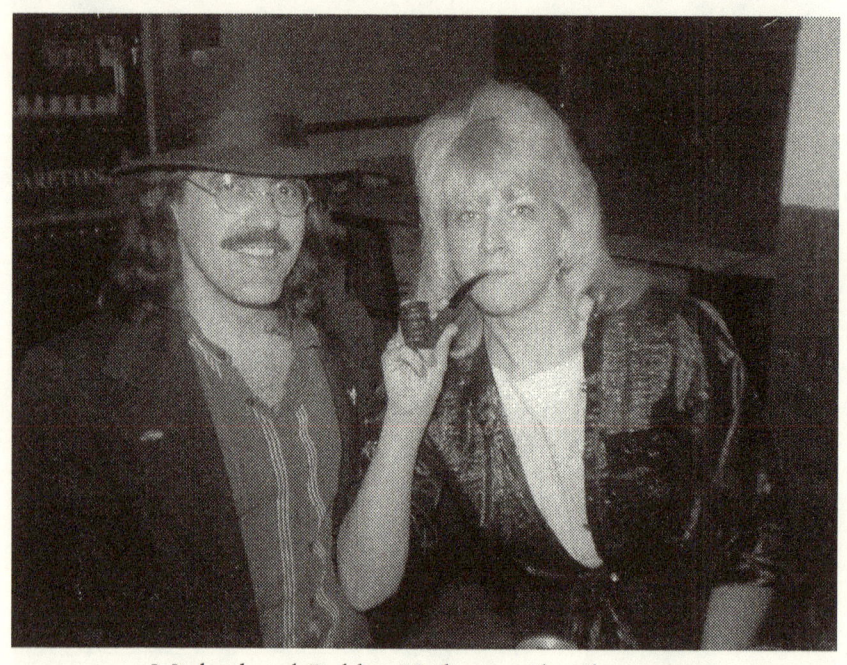

Michael and Debbie Hediger on break at a gig

Chapter 12
Blind Man on the River

My childhood memories of the Jack's Fork and Current River area are wonderful. I was spending quality time on those waterways before I was old enough to walk or talk.

When I was around thirteen my parents decided I was capable of floating the river alone. My father was an avid fisherman, and since I was readily available to guide his boat, I was given instruction at an early age.

The summer of 1964, at age fourteen, I was the skipper of a canoe during 27 trips from Alley Spring to Eminence, during which time the vessel capsized but once. This was, however, quite a monumental event since the canoe was folded in half, and my dad had to drag it from the river. (This event took place on the Jack's Fork River above Eminence, at the old railroad bridge.)

In 1968, my senior year, George Clark of Clark and Clark Drilling and I floated the upper Jack's Fork. George was a frequent customer at the Riverside Motel, which my parents owned at the time. George liked to drink, and of course, I would join him—not to do so would be alcohol abuse.

Apparently, I hadn't learned the art of pacing one's self, for before we were halfway to our destination I was sloshed. At one point I wrapped my canoe around a root wad. The canoe capsized and I was held under by the force of the rushing water. I couldn't move. I remember being able to see the sky from beneath the surface. I was beginning to panic when George yanked me from the water. It is a foregone conclusion that, if he hadn't been there, I wouldn't be here.

When we reached our destination darkness was approaching fast. George had his truck and I had mine. My young, brave, immature mind supposed I could make it home before being surrounded by total darkness. WRONG!

I had three problems. Number one, I was in unfamiliar territory; number two, I was drunk; and number three, the sun had gone down. To put it bluntly, I was blind. The antithesis of the proverbial vampire, I failed to return home before darkness prevailed.

Suddenly my fuzzy consciousness told me something wasn't right. The truck was running down a steep bank, and instead of hearing gravel beneath the tires, I heard leaves rustling and the sound of snapping tree limbs.

Miraculously, the truck safely came to a stop. I did what any blind drunk would do. I took a power nap.

I don't know how long I slept, but I was abruptly awakened by someone tapping on the window and a bright light in my eyes. The search party had found me.

They told me I had demolished a fence and rolled down an embankment. Just another day in the life of a blind hippie hillbilly!

During the late 70s, remembering the peace and solitude of floating the river alone, I decided it was time to relive the experience. Stocking a canoe with a 12-pack of beer I put in at Alley Spring with Eminence as my intended destination.

It was a beautiful, bright sunny day in the Ozark Mountains. Having grown up on the river, I had long ago learned to take only items absolutely necessary, for when (not if) the boat capsizes; the recovery of these items is a much simpler task.

With this thought in mind I would make the idiotic decision to leave my clear lenses behind. Why did I need them? It was a beautiful day. I could wear my prescription sunglasses.

About 30 minutes into the expedition the sun went bye-bye, and I took notice of an ominous cloud formation. I could see nothing but the surface of the water.

It was nerve-wracking. I couldn't panic. Knowing I must not lose control and give way to hysteria, I did the only thing I could do. I opened another beer.

On this day my skills at guiding a boat were quite useful. By observing the surface of the water as it reflected gray sky and hearing the sound of the flowing river, I was able to navigate the main stream.

It had begun to rain, making a bad situation worse. With drops of water on my sunglasses, I was almost totally blind.

Several hours, several miles, and several brews later, I was floating along in a daze, when I heard a faint voice calling my name. I thought it was an audio hallucination, but it wasn't. It was my mother.

With an instinct and love known only to a mother, she somehow sensed I was in trouble. I've always accused her of being too protective of me, but this time I was grateful.

To this day, I take great pride in my navigational skills. For many years I have found it amusing to watch tourists spinning their boats in circles as they attempt to float the river.

In 1994 I would guide a canoe down Current River for the last time. I was accompanied by two brave passengers, Debbie Hediger and her son Danny. It was a successful voyage, but I declared it to be my last, for it was no longer enjoyable. From this point forward I would let others do the driving.

However, at the conclusion of this final float trip, for which I was the guide, a notable event did take place. I would also fire a gun at a stationary target, never to do so again.

Hunting wasn't my thing, but having grown up around guns, they were quite familiar. I had learned to shoot before I could talk.

When we arrived at my dad's cabin after my final float trip, a shooting match was in progress.

As I watched I longed to take a shot at the target, which was a beer can about forty or fifty feet from the shooter. Each person was allowed three shots, standing, and without a rest. I took notice of the fact that not one person had hit the target shooting three shots consecutively.

Finally my dad said, "Son, do you think you can see well enough to hit the can?" With far too much pride, I stood up and said, "Sure."

My uncle, Harold McIntire, had been a shooting instructor in the military, and remembering his advise, I stood with my feet apart and toes pointed in for maximum stability. I could feel my pulse, and squeezing the trigger slowly between heartbeats, I fired the first round.

I could hardly see the can, but I saw it well enough to see it fly through the air. My second and third attempts were equally successful.

Feeling ten feet tall as I handed the pistol to my dad I realized this also would be a good day to conclude my shooting career.

I would have much the same experience while playing horseshoes for the last time. After taking at least five minutes I finally tossed the horseshoe, and as it spun around the stake I smiled to myself, for I knew this would be my final throw.

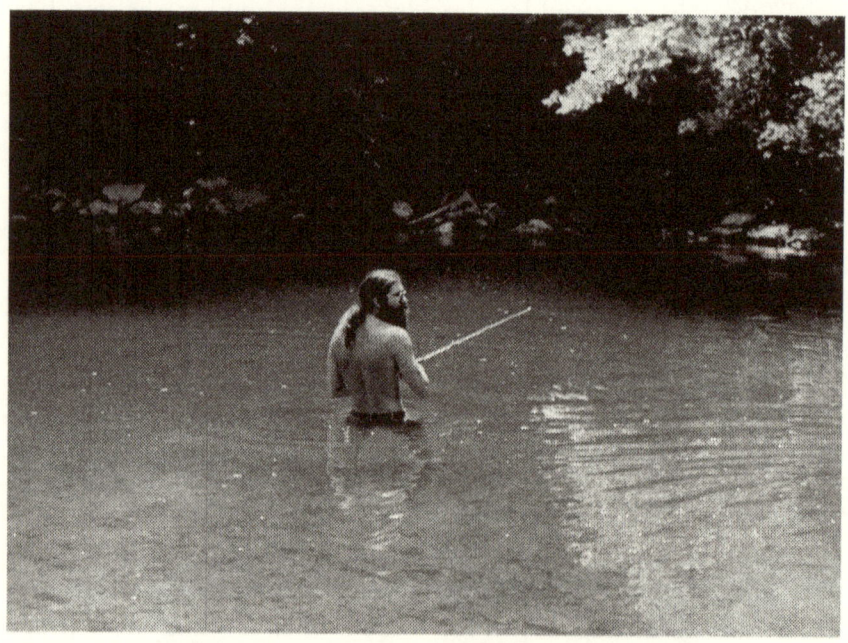

Michael fishing on the Current River (1980)

Chapter 13
Some Thoughts about Blindness

This will be my favorite chapter, because it will allow me to share my innermost thoughts and ideas concerning blindness. It's not as horrible as you may imagine. Since I once had sight, it's merely passing from one world to another. My memory, hearing, sense of touch, and sense of smell have never been better.

Sixty percent of our brain power is directed toward eyesight. If we lose this sense our brain power is simply transferred to our remaining senses.

For many years I would shine a light on my guitar while performing because I thought it necessary to see the neck. You will notice most guitarists are constantly looking at this part of the instrument while playing.

I was quite apprehensive the first night I performed without a light on my guitar, but by the end of the performance I was adapting, and during the weeks and months ahead I noticed a marked improvement.

Instead of using my eyes, I was using my ears. Not only was I a better musician, but my style of playing had changed. In other words, I left one world and entered another. This has not only been the case in music, but in every aspect of my life.

As I have grown older, I find it interesting to observe people's reaction to my blindness. I am aware of patience being a virtue, but I don't suffer fools well.

For instance, several times as I toured the country some good old boy would say to me, "I don't know how you can stand being blind. I couldn't handle that." Finally, upon having this said to me in Everett, Washington, while taking a break during a performance, my response was swift.

I said, "I'd rather be blind than stupid." I now have a t-shirt stating this opinion in large, black, bold letters. However, the joke's probably on me, for a person making a statement such as this would likely be unable to read.

I remember an incident in the mid-70's, when the Blind Association visited my home in Springfield, Missouri. They immediately tried to categorize me as being the poor pitiful blind boy. After an eternity of stupid questions, my pleasant personality dwindled.

Finally, when they asked my denomination of faith, not understanding what this had to do with blindness, I snapped, "I tried them all, but I still can't see."

I love it when someone says, "You don't look blind." What the hell do you say to an idiotic statement such as this? After giving it some thought, I finally came up with an appropriate response. I simply ask, "What does a blind person look like?" Man, you've never heard such stuttering and stammering. I've yet to receive an answer.

I do, however, understand their meaning. I do a pretty good imitation of Stevie Wonder, flashing his teeth and swaying to and fro. I might roll my eyes back in my head and take my sunglasses off, asking if this is what a blind man looks like. Sometimes I just can't resist being a smartass.

Speaking of sunglasses, in the year 2000, we had been playing a bar in Bullhead City, Arizona, and had been there several weeks, when I was informed of several patrons sporting sunglasses on a regular basis. I found this to be amusing, since they most certainly thought I was just trying to be cool.

I try, but it's hard to be cool when you can't see. I do, however, have the advantage, for I once had sight so most of the time I can keep the awkwardness to a minimum, unless I take a drink and the straw sticks in my nostril, or I fall off the stage. Then so much for Mr. Cool!

Speaking of Mr. Cool, many times through the years I would be performing my little heart out when abruptly there would be a prodigious amount of applause. Glowing with excitement I would gratefully thank the audience only to find, much to my consternation, that they were applauding a good pool shot or a seductive move on the dance floor.

The standing ovations I've received during my career may be counted on one hand. I was not informed of those memorable occasions until days or weeks after their occurrence, which is probably a good thing, for I would have had to purchase a new hat.

Sometimes the shoe would be on the other foot. Beautiful insecure women, craving attention, would wiggle and jiggle in front of me while I was playing guitar, totally oblivious of their seductive actions. For some strange reason, my girlfriends always found this delightful.

Some women cannot accept my inability to visualize their beauty, so they resort to desperate measures. They have actually taken my hands and run them over their face and body, hoping this would present a clear picture in my mind.

It is, however, quite impossible to enjoy such activities to their full capacity, knowing at any moment that seeing stars is an option, if your girlfriend happens to glance your way.

In 1996 I was asked to judge a short-skirt contest while performing at Ramone's in Springfield. It was during the recording of my CD *Live at Ramone's,* and there were around 300 people in the house. Thirty anxious ladies were awaiting my decision. Sounds like fun doesn't it? I can promise you, if I had been feeling bare legs I would still be reminiscing, but this was not to be the case, for there is nothing sexy about the feel of synthetic material. Being the consummate entertainer I played my assigned role for all it was worth and everyone had a good laugh.

A person's reaction to my perceived handicap speaks volumes about his or her character. All I have to do is read the signs. Some are very attentive while others don't have a clue, nor do they care. We don't want pity, but a little understanding is welcome.

Some are far too protective, but I'll take this over apathy. Most people care. That's the bottom line. Maybe the average citizen is unaware of a blind person's needs, but the majority is willing to learn.

There are approximately 8800 people in Shannon County, where I now reside. Blind people are few and far between in them thar hills. To my knowledge there are only three of us, so it is perfectly reasonable to assume a lack of experience when others attempt to meet our particular needs.

This problem, however, is universal. People have waved hello and goodbye to me in no less than two thirds of the states in America, and I have yet to be aware of it until someone reminds them of my situation. I wear sunglasses in public while being guided by another person, and they still don't get it. They look without seeing.

It can be both humorous and frustrating. For instance, when I ask the location of an object in a room the typical response is, "It's over there." They describe the object as a thing. I try to be patient. It's a constant effort to educate people of my situation.

The blind must have details such as direction, distance, description of objects, etc.

As my sight is diminished I am forced to become organized. I recommend this to everyone. Before I completely lost my sight I spent most of my life looking for misplaced items. Yes, it's true. Now that I can't see I know where most things are. That's when the memory kicks in. If the memory goes, it's all over. Take me to the nearest nursing home.

Rule number 1 in Michael's house: Return items to their proper place after use. Some of my friends find it quite amusing to rearrange the furniture while I'm away from home.

Rule number 2: Don't booby trap the blind man. Many times I have found myself in agony after falling over a vacuum cleaner left in the middle of the floor. They always apologize, but I swear I can sometimes hear snickering in the next room. Throwing dirty laundry on the basement steps can also be hazardous to my health.

Rule number 3: Please don't put bathroom cleaner in place of my mouth wash container. (This has actually happened to me.)

I find it impossible to understand why people shout at me. They yell as if I'm on the next ridge rather than in the same room. I tell them I'm blind, not deaf, but they continue to shout.

While they're shouting at you they sometimes describe the clothes you're wearing, as if you didn't know. He's blind. He must be an idiot.

I have experienced very little prejudice because of my blindness. I believe this is due, in part, to my lifestyle. Certainly, I could not make this claim, if I had been an active member of the 9-to-5 work force.

Nothing could be considered normal in the music world. In fact, there is a greater tolerance of the abnormal.

Many subscribe to the myth that blind people make better music. If this is so, it's probably because they would most likely hear their mistakes. The concept of playing music is simple. If it doesn't sound good, don't play it.

Amazingly, I depend a great deal on my remaining sight. As I walk through my home I use lamps and the light from windows as a beacon. This allows me to remain aware of my location in the room with each step I take. My point is this. Utilize your senses no matter how diminished they may be.

People look, but they don't see. Recently I was thinking of taking a walk on the road from my house to the highway. Knowing my housekeeper had driven the road but a few minutes earlier, I asked if there were puddles in the road. She told me she didn't know.

This is hard for me to comprehend, for in my world you would definitely hear the vehicle pass through the puddles. When I was in the sighted world I was also guilty of this crime. If my vision were restored tomorrow I wonder how long it would be before I too would look without seeing.

I am frequently approached by people who ask the question, "Do you know who I am?" Okay. I get it. They want to know if I recognize their voice. Relying upon the full powers of my wit, I devised a retort. I simply smile and say, "If you don't know who you are, then how the hell would I know?"

Some people have a very distinctive voice. My hometown buddy Jimmy Caylor loves to tell this story. I hadn't been home for many years, and seated in a crowded, noisy bar, I could hear Jimmy's voice across the bar. With my back to him I yelled his name quite loudly. I knew what I was doing, and as I sat there smiling, he spent several minutes trying to ascertain my location. Isn't it ironic, that after all the years of not having been in each other's company, the blind home boy knew who he was, but he didn't recognize me? I'm sure my hair being three feet shorter than the last time he saw me had absolutely nothing to do with it.

Often when I meet a person I will recognize their voice for the remainder of my life, but this is not the norm. In most instances I must become familiar with a person's voice before making a connection.

I suppose it's because I'm a grandpa rock'n'roller, but I have the greatest problem identifying the voices of people in their twenties and thirties, or should I say the MTV generation. Their voices are indistinguishable to me. Maybe someone should put some acid in their bubblegum. Just kidding!

Being disabled has sharpened my vision of human nature. Quite frankly, experience has taught me that if people are uncomfortable in my presence because of my blindness, or are inconsiderate, then they are shallow human beings, and this hippie hillbilly long-haired songster should avoid associating with them by all means.

I have also become adept at recognizing warm, caring, sensitive human beings, and relationships with these people will inevitably make a better person of me.

Everyone should strive to surround themselves with trustworthy, loyal, and sincere people, but man, if you're blind; you'd better place this at the top of your to-do list.

Like everything else in my life I had to learn about women the hard way, but by the time I reached thirty, it began to slowly sink in. When searching for the right mate, luck is definitely a factor, but a little knowledge and wisdom can be quite beneficial.

To illustrate, sharing with you my first encounter with the love of my life, Sandie Zemblidge, is in order. Living in the woods alone and blind I realized that if I was to meet a woman with whom I was compatible I would have to take the initiative, so I joined an online dating service.

Two weeks after joining, and after receiving several messages which were quite laughable, if not sad, first contact was made.

Sandie's message illuminated the darkness. Within a few paragraphs I knew there was gold in them thar hills. During our first conversation we fell in love. I sent her to my web site (blind-cat.com) knowing she would learn of my blindness.

We've been together for 18 months, so I suppose the question of whether or not this would be an issue was answered. She is a person always putting others before herself. I learn from her on a daily basis.

Recently Sandie has been in my dreams, and much to my chagrin, she is without a face. I have a picture in my mind of her, but for the first time in my life I'm having a relationship with a woman I've never seen.

If you'll pardon the pun, I was blind-sided by the dreams, for this was something I'd not thought of. My dreams are quite normal, if they pertain to something in my past, but if they're about something I haven't seen, my imagination kicks in.

I would be curious to know what a person being blind from birth sees in their dreams.

Through the years I've experienced a wide range of reactions from the parents whose daughter I would be involved with at the time. Consisting of everything from shock to total acceptance

The most common question asked of these women is, "Why would you want to date a blind man?"

This leads me to my next topic. SEX! Don't worry. I'll keep it clean. They say something good always comes from something bad. I see with my hands, so it stands to reason my sense of touch would be acute. In other words, baby, I got the magic touch. Please! No cards and letters.

Curiosity is natural, so when the girls at the office ask Sandie personal questions she merely smiles and says, "There's nothing like the touch of a blind man."

I'm sure I discover things other people would overlook. Once upon a time I met a lady with webbed toes. I'm not lying; she was webbed between her second and third toe on both feet. She told me I was the first to discover this fact.

Here's some advice for the ladies out there. If you sometimes miss a spot shaving your legs, or if you've got hair on your toes or other abnormalities, beware of blind men. Remember! I can tell if you're fat or thin with no more than a simple hand shake.

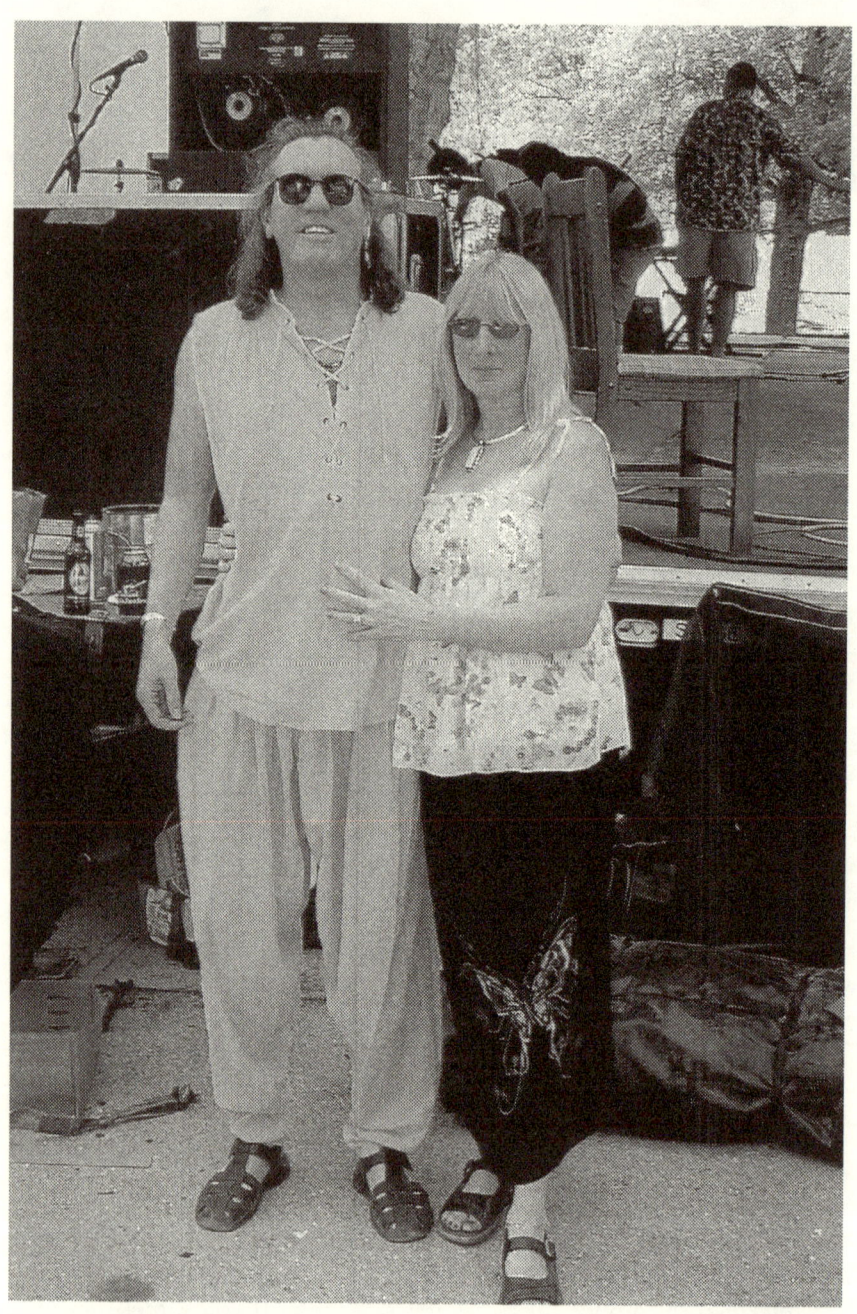

Michael and Sandie after his performance at Schwagfest 2005

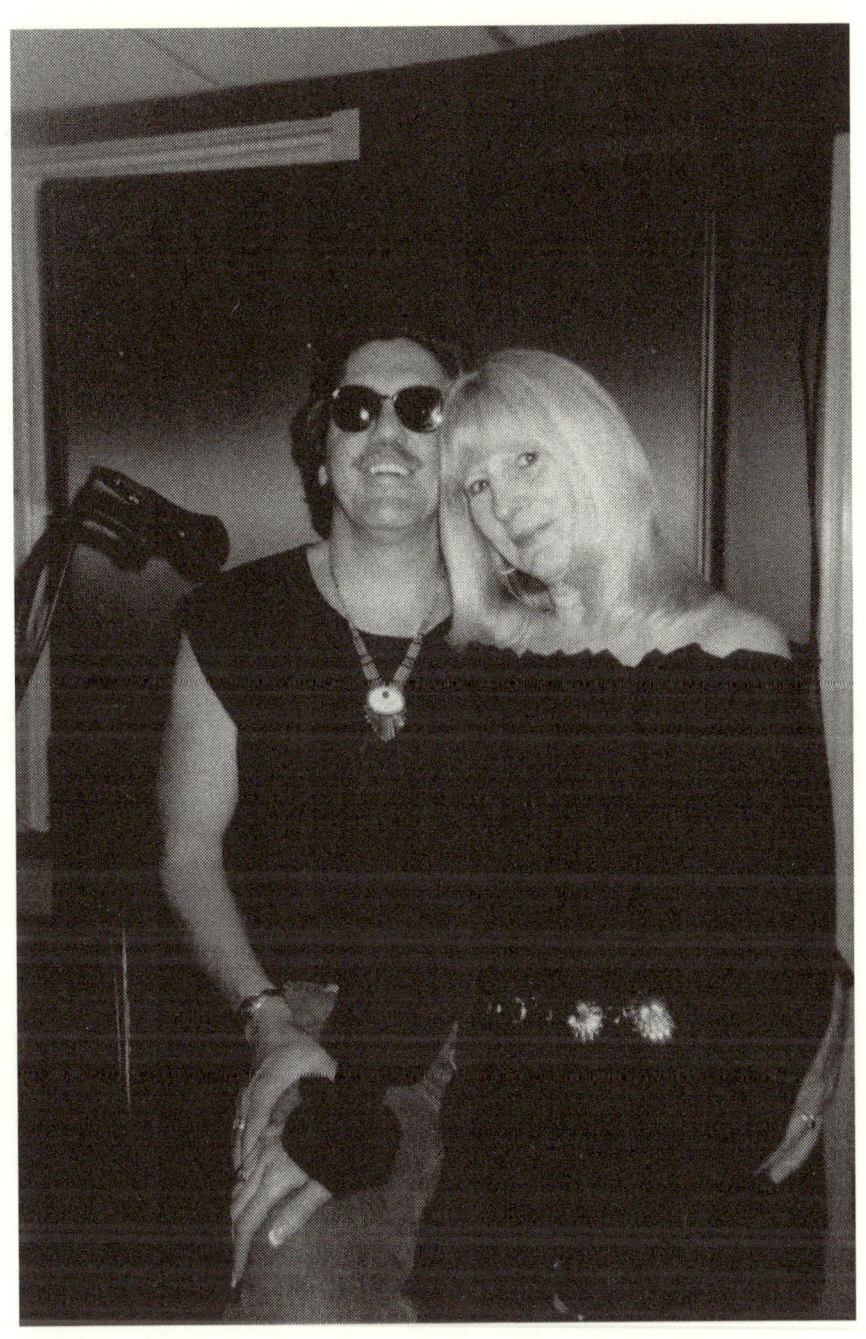

Michael and Sandie on break at Rube's Roost 2003

Chapter 14
Last Vestige of Sight

As the lights dim and I pass into a world of darkness, being only able to see the flicker of a candle, or the sun on a bright day, I do so without fear, for I am surrounded by love. Ray Charles is quoted as saying, "Eyesight is only one percent of life." Each day I strive to love and learn.

We are dealt a hand of cards, and how those cards are played is our choice to make. When God dealt my hand the cards consisted of health, stunning looks, talent, intelligence, creativity, wisdom, and oh yeah — did I forget to include modesty? He must have looked at my hand and thought, "Hmmmmmmmm! This looks too good I'd better throw in a joker."

I strongly believe in the power of positive thinking, while entering into a new and exciting world. Of course I miss gazing into the faces of my friends and loved ones, especially my daughters and Sandie, but there is a positive side to this coin.

When I hear the voices of my parents or old friends I see their faces as they were thirty years ago. They are ageless. I like the idea of never looking into a mirror and seeing an old man staring back at me.

As I live the remainder of my days in the Ozark Mountains, I miss being able to gaze across the majestic hills or experience the scenery of the river from a canoe, but I just can't bring myself to whine about it, for I was once able to see the wonders of the world. In my view the glass is always half full.

I have seen the best of what life has to offer, and these memories are forever programmed deep within my soul. These eyes have gazed upon colorful sunsets, '57 Chevys, Harley Davidsons, the perfection of the female form and most precious of all, the faces of my beautiful twin daughters, Dillan Margot and Dane Michael. What could I possibly have to cry about? It has been, and continues to be, a wonderful and exciting life.

The end

Blind Jokes

- At The Airport

The entrance opens, two men dressed in pilots' uniforms walk up the aisle. Both are wearing dark glasses, one is using a guide dog, and the other is tapping his way along the aisle with a cane. Nervous laughter spreads through the cabin, but the men enter the cockpit, the door closes, and the engines start up.

The passengers begin glancing nervously around, searching for some sign that this is just a little practical joke. None is forthcoming. The plane moves faster and faster down the runway, and the people sitting in the window seats realize they're headed straight for the water at the edge of the airport property. As it begins to look as though the plane will plow into the water, panicked screams fill the cabin. At that moment, the plane lifts smoothly into the air. The passengers relax and laugh a little sheepishly, and soon all retreat into their magazines, secure in the knowledge that the plane is in good hands.

In the cockpit, one of the blind pilots turns to the other and says, "You know, Frank, one of these days, they're gonna scream too late and we're all gonna die."

- Ethnic Idiosyncrasies

A blind man and his guide dog enter a bar and find their way to a barstool. After ordering a drink, and sitting there for a while, the blind guy yells to the bartender, "Hey, you wanna hear a blonde joke ?" The bar immediately becomes absolutely quiet. In a husky, deep voice, the woman next to him says, "Before you tell that joke, you should know something. The bartender is blonde, the bouncer is blonde, and I'm a 6' tall, 200 lb. blonde with a black belt in karate. What's more, the woman sitting next to me is blonde and she's a weight lifter. The lady to your right is a blonde, and she's a wrestler. Think about it seriously, Mister. You still wanna tell that joke?" The blind guy says, "Nah, not if I'm gonna have to explain it five times."

- Legal Tango

A police department famous for its superior canine (K-9) unit was somewhat taken back by a recent incident. Returning home from work a blonde was shocked to find her house ransacked and burglarized. She telephoned the police to report the crime. The dispatcher broadcast the call on the radio and it happened that a K9 unit was on foot patrol nearby. As the officer approaches, his dog on a leash the blonde emerges from the house, claps a hand to her head and moans, "I come home from work to find all my possessions stolen. I call the police for help and they send me a blind cop?!?"

- And Then There Was The ...

...blind man who went into a store with his seeing eye dog. After a few minutes he takes the leash and swings the dog over and around his head. The manager comes over and yells. "Just what do you think you are doing?!?" The blind man calmly replied, "Oh, just looking around."

- Religious Hygiene

A nun in a convent walks into the bathroom where Sister Patrice is taking a shower. "A blind man is here to see you," she reported "Well, if he's blind it doesn't matter that I'm in the shower. Show him in." The man walks into the room and the Sister tells him how very much they appreciate all the work he does at the convent. For 10 minutes she goes on about the jobs. Finally, he interrupts and say,"That's very nice, ma'ma but you can put your clothes back on now and tell me ... where do you want these blinds?"

–Gone To The Dogs

A man goes into a bar with his dog. He walks up to the bar and orders a drink. "You can't bring a dog in here", the bartender tells him. The guy, without missing a beat says, "sorry, but this is my seeing eye dog." "Oh man!", the bartender exclaims. "Here have the first one on me." The guy graciously accepts the drink and walks to a table near the door. A second man comes in with a small Chihuahua. The first man stops him and says "they won't serve you unless you tell the barkeep that your dog is a seeing eye dog." Thanking the guy, the second guy walks to the bar and orders a drink. "You can't bring your dog in the bar, sir." "But, he's my seeing eye dog," the guy explains. "Don't give me that," the bartender tells him. "They don't use Chihuahua's for seeing eye dogs!' The guy pauses for a second and muses, "They gave me a Chihuahua?"

–The Fragrance Department

A woman goes into Wal-Mart to buy a rod and reel for her grandson's birthday She doesn't know which one to get so she just grabs one and goes over to the counter. A Wal-Mart associate is standing there wearing dark shades. She says, "Excuse me, sir. Can you tell me anything about this rod and reel?"

He says, "Ma'am, I'm completely blind; but if you'll drop it on the counter, I can tell you everything you need to know about it from the sound it makes. She doesn't believe him but drops it on the counter anyway. He says, "That's a six-foot Shakespeare graphite rod with a Zebco 404 reel and 10-pound test line. It's a good all around combination; and it's on sale this week for only $20.00." She says, "It's amazing that you can tell all that just by the sound of it dropping on the counter. I'll take it!" As she opens her purse, her credit card drops on the floor. "Oh, that sounds like a Visa card," he says. She bends down to pick it up and accidentally breaks wind. At first she is really embarrassed, but then realizes there is no way the blind clerk could tell it was she who farted. Being blind, he wouldn't know that she was the only person around.

The man rings up the sale and says, "That'll be $34.50 plus tax." The woman is totally confused by this and asks, "Didn't you tell me it was on sale for $20.00? How did you get $34.50?" He replies, "Yes, Ma'am. The rod and reel is $20.00, but the Duck Call is $11.00 and the Catfish Bait is $3.50."

-Tee For Two

This golfer had lost his sight over the years, but just refused to give in and not be able to play, so the golf pro said there was an older gentleman that had gotten feeble and couldn't swing a club anymore but had tremendous sight. So the blind guy said, "That is great; that way they both could stay with the game." So on the first tee, the older gentleman tees the ball up for the blind player and positions him. He swings and hits it good. The gentleman says, "mister that was a good hit." The blind man says, Where did it go?" The older gentleman answers, "I don't know, I forgot."

- "I was in the library and fell asleep. When I woke up, a blind man was reading my face. I get no respect." - Rodney Dangerfield.

-The Bus Ride

A husband and wife are waiting at the bus stop, and with them are their nine children.

A blind man joins them after a few minutes. When the bus arrives, they find it overloaded and only the wife and the nine kids are able to fit in the bus.

So the husband and the blind man decide to walk. After a while the husband gets irritated by the ticking of the stick of the blind man as he taps it on the side walk and says to him: "Why don't you put a piece of rubber at the end your stick, that ticking sound is driving me crazy!" The blind man replies: "If you would've put a rubber on the end of YOUR stick, we'd be riding the bus, so shut the hell up!"

About the Author

Michael McIntire is an accomplished musician, and has entertained throughout the United States, spanning a career of forty two years. His music being eclectic includes rock, country, blues, and bluegrass. He plays the guitar, banjo, harmonica, and violin.

Michael has recorded four music c.d.'s titled; Runnin Wild, 1982, Live at Ramone's 1996, Live 2000, and Back to Current River, 2003. In his most recent c.d., Back to Current River, he wrote, produced, vocalized, and recorded all instruments except dobro.

In his latest creative endeavor as the author of Blind Man Running, he adds another perspective to his life as a blind musician, not only telling his story with song, but with the written word.

Michael lives in the beautiful Ozark Mountains, in south central Missouri, with his lady, Sandie.

Visit Michael's web site, at blind-cat.com

www.ingramcontent.com/pod-product-compliance
Lightning Source LLC
Chambersburg PA
CBHW020247290526
45784CB00003B/1141